Fungal Infection

DIAGNOSIS
AND MANAGEMENT

Fungal Infection

DIAGNOSIS

AND MANAGEMENT

Malcolm D. Richardson

BSc, PhD, CBiol, MIBiol, FRCPath
Consultant Clinical Scientist in Mycology
Regional Mycology Reference Laboratory
Department of Dermatology
University of Glasgow and
West Glasgow Hospitals University NHS Trust
Glasgow

David W. Warnock

BSc, PhD, CBiol, FIBiol, FRCPath
Consultant Clinical Scientist in Mycology
Mycology Reference Laboratory
Public Health Laboratory Service
Bristol

SECOND EDITION

Blackwell
Science

© 1993, 1997 by
Blackwell Science Ltd
Editorial Offices:
Osney Mead, Oxford OX2 0EL
25 John Street, London WC1N 2BL
23 Ainslie Place, Edinburgh EH3 6AJ
350 Main Street, Malden
  MA 02148 5018, USA
54 University Street, Carlton
  Victoria 3053, Australia

Other Editorial Offices:
Blackwell Wissenschafts-Verlag GmbH
Kurfürstendamm 57
10707 Berlin, Germany

Zehetnergasse 6
1140 Wien, Austria

First published 1993
Reprinted 1994 (twice)
Second edition 1997

Set by DP Photosetting, Aylesbury, Bucks
Printed and bound in Great Britain
by Hartnolls Ltd, Bodmin, Cornwall

DISTRIBUTORS

Marston Book Services Ltd
PO Box 269
Abingdon, Oxon OX14 4YN
(*Orders:* Tel: 01235 465500
        Fax: 01235 465555)
USA
Blackwell Science, Inc.
Commerce Place
350 Main Street
Malden, MA 02148 5018
(*Orders:* Tel: 800 759 6102
        617 388 8250
     Fax: 617 388 8255)
Canada
Copp Clark Professional
200 Adelaide St West, 3rd Floor
Toronto, Ontario M5H 1W7
(*Orders:* Tel: 416 597-1616
        800 815-9417
     Fax: 416 597-1617)
Australia
Blackwell Science Pty Ltd
54 University Street
Carlton, Victoria 3053
(*Orders:* Tel: 3 9347 0300
     Fax: 3 9347 5001)

A catalogue record for this title
is available from the British Library

ISBN 0-86542-724-0

Library of Congress
Cataloging-in-publication Data

Richardson, M. D.
  Fungal infection : diagnosis and
  management / Malcolm D. Richardson,
  David W. Warnock. 2nd ed.
     p.   cm.
  Includes bibliographical references and
index.
  ISBN 0-86542-724-0
  1. Mycoses. I. Warnock, D. W. II. Title.
  [DNLM: 1. Mycoses–diagnosis.
  2. Mycoses–therapy. WC 450 R524f 1997]
  RC117.R47 1997
  616.9'69–DC21   97-5802
                                     CIP

Contents

Preface to the second edition, xix
Preface to the first edition, xx
Acknowledgements, xxi

1 Introduction, 1
1.1 The nature of fungi, 1
1.2 Fungi as human pathogens, 2
    1.2.1 The superficial mycoses, 3
    1.2.2 The subcutaneous mycoses, 3
    1.2.3 The systemic mycoses, 4
1.3 The changing pattern of fungal infection, 5
1.4 Implications for diagnosis and management, 7

2 Laboratory diagnosis of fungal infection, 9
2.1 Introduction, 9
2.2 Collection of specimens, 10
    2.2.1 Skin, nails and hair, 10
    2.2.2 Mucous membranes, 11
    2.2.3 Ear, 11
    2.2.4 Eye, 12
    2.2.5 Blood, 12
    2.2.6 Cerebrospinal fluid, 13
    2.2.7 Urine, 13
    2.2.8 Other fluids, 13
    2.2.9 Lower respiratory tract specimens, 13
    2.2.10 Pus, 14
    2.2.11 Bone marrow, 14
    2.2.12 Tissue, 15
2.3 Specimens for serological tests, 15
2.4 Specimens for antifungal drug level determinations, 15
2.5 Transport of specimens, 15
2.6 Interpretation of laboratory test results, 16
    2.6.1 Direct microscopic examination, 16
    2.6.2 Culture, 17
    2.6.3 Serological tests, 18
    2.6.4 Histopathological examination, 18

3 Antifungal drugs, 20
3.1 Introduction, 20

3.2 Amphotericin B, 20
    3.2.1   Mechanism of action, 20
    3.2.2   Spectrum of action, 21
    3.2.3   Acquired resistance, 21
    3.2.4   Pharmacokinetics, 21
    3.2.5   Metabolism, 23
    3.2.6   Pharmaceutics, 23
    3.2.7   Therapeutic use, 24
    3.2.8   Mode of administration, 25
    3.2.9   Adverse reactions, 28
    3.2.10 Drug interactions, 30
3.3 Fluconazole, 30
    3.3.1   Mechanism of action, 30
    3.3.2   Spectrum of action, 30
    3.3.3   Acquired resistance, 31
    3.3.4   Pharmacokinetics, 31
    3.3.5   Metabolism, 32
    3.3.6   Pharmaceutics, 32
    3.3.7   Therapeutic use, 32
    3.3.8   Mode of administration, 33
    3.3.9   Adverse reactions, 34
    3.3.10 Drug interactions, 34
3.4 Flucytosine, 35
    3.4.1   Mechanism of action, 35
    3.4.2   Spectrum of action, 35
    3.4.3   Acquired resistance, 36
    3.4.4   Pharmacokinetics, 36
    3.4.5   Metabolism, 36
    3.4.6   Pharmaceutics, 37
    3.4.7   Therapeutic use, 37
    3.4.8   Mode of administration, 37
    3.4.9   Adverse reactions, 37
    3.4.10 Drug interactions, 38
3.5 Griseofulvin, 38
    3.5.1   Mechanism of action, 38
    3.5.2   Spectrum of action, 39
    3.5.3   Acquired resistance, 39
    3.5.4   Pharmacokinetics, 39
    3.5.5   Metabolism, 39
    3.5.6   Pharmaceutics, 39
    3.5.7   Therapeutic use, 39
    3.5.8   Mode of administration, 40
    3.5.9   Adverse reactions, 40
    3.5.10 Drug interactions, 40
3.6 Itraconazole, 40
    3.6.1   Mechanism of action, 40
    3.6.2   Spectrum of action, 41

3.6.3   Acquired resistance, 41
3.6.4   Pharmacokinetics, 41
3.6.5   Metabolism, 42
3.6.6   Pharmaceutics, 42
3.6.7   Therapeutic use, 42
3.6.8   Mode of administration, 42
3.6.9   Adverse reactions, 43
3.6.10   Drug interactions, 44
3.7   Ketoconazole, 44
3.7.1   Mechanism of action, 45
3.7.2   Spectrum of action, 45
3.7.3   Acquired resistance, 45
3.7.4   Pharmacokinetics, 45
3.7.5   Metabolism, 45
3.7.6   Pharmaceutics, 45
3.7.7   Therapeutic use, 46
3.7.8   Mode of administration, 46
3.7.9   Adverse reactions, 46
3.7.10   Drug interactions, 47
3.8   Miconazole, 47
3.8.1   Mechanism of action, 47
3.8.2   Spectrum of action, 48
3.8.3   Acquired resistance, 48
3.8.4   Pharmacokinetics, 48
3.8.5   Metabolism, 48
3.8.6   Pharmaceutics, 48
3.8.7   Therapeutic use, 49
3.8.8   Mode of administration, 49
3.8.9   Adverse reactions, 49
3.8.10   Drug interactions, 50
3.9   Terbinafine, 50
3.9.1   Mechanism of action, 50
3.9.2   Spectrum of action, 50
3.9.3   Acquired resistance, 50
3.9.4   Pharmacokinetics, 50
3.9.5   Metabolism, 51
3.9.6   Pharmaceutics, 51
3.9.7   Therapeutic use, 51
3.9.8   Mode of administration, 51
3.9.9   Adverse reactions, 52
3.9.10   Drug interactions, 52
3.10   Other compounds for topical administration, 52
3.10.1   Amorolfine, 52
3.10.2   Bifonazole, 52
3.10.3   Clotrimazole, 52
3.10.4   Econazole nitrate, 53
3.10.5   Isoconazole nitrate, 53

3.10.6   Naftifine, 53
3.10.7   Natamycin, 53
3.10.8   Nystatin, 53
3.10.9   Sulconazole nitrate, 53
3.10.10   Tioconazole, 53
3.11 Empirical treatment of suspected fungal infection in the neutropenic patient, 53
3.12 Prophylactic treatment for prevention of fungal infection, 54
3.13 Laboratory monitoring, 55
     3.13.1   Amphotericin B, 55
     3.13.2   Fluconazole, 56
     3.13.3   Flucytosine, 57
     3.13.4   Itraconazole, 57
     3.13.5   Ketoconazole, 58

4 Dermatophytosis, 59
4.1 Introduction, 59
4.2 The causal organisms and their habitat, 59
4.3 Laboratory diagnosis of dermatophytosis, 60
4.4 Tinea capitis, 61
     4.4.1   Definition, 61
     4.4.2   Geographical distribution, 61
     4.4.3   Causal organisms, 61
     4.4.4   Clinical manifestations, 62
     4.4.5   Differential diagnosis, 63
     4.4.6   Essential investigations and their interpretation, 63
     4.4.7   Management, 64
4.5 Tinea corporis, 65
     4.5.1   Definition, 65
     4.5.2   Geographical distribution, 65
     4.5.3   Causal organisms, 65
     4.5.4   Clinical manifestations, 65
     4.5.5   Differential diagnosis, 66
     4.5.6   Essential investigations and their interpretation, 66
     4.5.7   Management, 66
4.6 Tinea cruris, 67
     4.6.1   Definition, 67
     4.6.2   Geographical distribution, 67
     4.6.3   Causal organisms, 67
     4.6.4   Clinical manifestations, 67
     4.6.5   Differential diagnosis, 68
     4.6.6   Essential investigations and their interpretation, 68
     4.6.7   Management, 68

4.7 Tinea pedis, 69
   4.7.1 Definition, 69
   4.7.2 Geographical distribution, 69
   4.7.3 Causal organisms, 69
   4.7.4 Clinical manifestations, 69
   4.7.5 Differential diagnosis, 70
   4.7.6 Essential investigations and their interpretation, 71
   4.7.7 Management, 71
4.8 Tinea manuum, 72
   4.8.1 Definition, 72
   4.8.2 Geographical distribution, 72
   4.8.3 Causal organisms, 72
   4.8.4 Clinical manifestations, 73
   4.8.5 Differential diagnosis, 73
   4.8.6 Essential investigations and their interpretation, 74
   4.8.7 Management, 74
4.9 Tinea unguium, 74
   4.9.1 Definition, 74
   4.9.2 Geographical distribution, 74
   4.9.3 Causal organisms, 74
   4.9.4 Clinical manifestations, 75
   4.9.5 Differential diagnosis, 75
   4.9.6 Essential investigations and their interpretation, 76
   4.9.7 Management, 77

5 Superficial candidosis, 78
5.1 Definition, 78
5.2 Geographical distribution, 78
5.3 The causal organisms and their habitat, 78
5.4 Clinical manifestations, 79
   5.4.1 Oral candidosis, 79
   5.4.2 Vaginal candidosis, 81
   5.4.3 Penile candidosis, 82
   5.4.4 Cutaneous candidosis, 83
   5.4.5 *Candida* nail infection, 84
   5.4.6 Chronic mucocutaneous candidosis, 85
5.5 Superficial candidosis in special hosts, 86
5.6 Essential investigations and their interpretation, 87
5.7 Management, 87
   5.7.1 Oral candidosis, 87
   5.7.2 Vaginal candidosis, 89
   5.7.3 Penile candidosis, 91
   5.7.4 Cutaneous candidosis, 92
   5.7.5 *Candida* nail infection, 92

5.7.6   Chronic mucocutaneous candidosis, 92

6 Other cutaneous fungal infections, 94
6.1   Pityriasis versicolor, 94
    6.1.1   Definition, 94
    6.1.2   Geographical distribution, 94
    6.1.3   The causal organism and its habitat, 94
    6.1.4   Clinical manifestations, 95
    6.1.5   Differential diagnosis, 95
    6.1.6   Essential investigations and their interpretation, 96
    6.1.7   Management, 96
6.2   Other *Malassezia* infections, 97
    6.2.1   *Malassezia* folliculitis, 97
    6.2.2   Seborrhoeic dermatitis, 97
6.3   Piedra, 98
6.4   White piedra, 98
    6.4.1   Definition, 98
    6.4.2   Geographical distribution, 98
    6.4.3   The causal organism and its habitat, 99
    6.4.4   Clinical manifestations, 99
    6.4.5   Differential diagnosis, 99
    6.4.6   Essential investigations and their interpretation, 99
    6.4.7   Management, 100
6.5   Black piedra, 100
    6.5.1   Definition, 100
    6.5.2   Geographical distribution, 100
    6.5.3   The causal organism and its habitat, 100
    6.5.4   Clinical manifestations, 100
    6.5.5   Differential diagnosis, 101
    6.5.6   Essential investigations and their interpretation, 101
    6.5.7   Management, 101
6.6   Tinea nigra, 101
    6.6.1   Definition, 101
    6.6.2   Geographical distribution, 101
    6.6.3   The causal organism and its habitat, 101
    6.6.4   Clinical manifestations, 102
    6.6.5   Differential diagnosis, 102
    6.6.6   Essential investigations and their interpretation, 102
    6.6.7   Management, 102
6.7   *Scytalidium* infection, 102

7 Mould infections of nails, 104
7.1   Definition, 104

7.2 Geographical distribution, 104
7.3 The causal organisms and their habitat, 104
7.4 Clinical manifestations, 105
7.5 Differential diagnosis, 105
7.6 Essential investigations and their interpretation, 105
7.7 Management, 106

8 Keratomycosis, 107
8.1 Definition, 107
8.2 Geographical distribution, 107
8.3 The causal organisms and their habitat, 107
8.4 Clinical manifestations, 108
8.5 Essential investigations and their interpretation, 108
8.6 Management, 109

9 Otomycosis, 111
9.1 Definition, 111
9.2 Geographical distribution, 111
9.3 The causal organisms and their habitat, 111
9.4 Clinical manifestations, 111
9.5 Differential diagnosis, 112
9.6 Essential investigations and their interpretation, 112
9.7 Management, 112

10 Aspergillosis, 113
10.1 Definition, 113
10.2 Geographical distribution, 113
10.3 The causal organisms and their habitat, 113
10.4 Clinical manifestations, 114
    10.4.1 Allergic aspergillosis, 114
    10.4.2 Fungus ball of the lung, 115
    10.4.3 Chronic necrotizing aspergillosis of the lung, 115
    10.4.4 Acute invasive aspergillosis of the lung, 116
    10.4.5 Tracheobronchitis and obstructing bronchial aspergillosis, 117
    10.4.6 Sinusitis, 117
    10.4.7 Cerebral aspergillosis, 118
    10.4.8 Ocular aspergillosis, 119
    10.4.9 Endocarditis and myocarditis, 119
    10.4.10 Osteomyelitis, 120
    10.4.11 Cutaneous aspergillosis, 120
    10.4.12 Other forms of aspergillosis, 121
10.5 Aspergillosis in special hosts, 121
    10.5.1 Patients with AIDS, 121
10.6 Essential investigations and their interpretation, 122
    10.6.1 Microscopy, 122

10.6.2   Culture, 123
10.6.3   Skin tests, 123
10.6.4   Serological tests, 123
10.7 Management, 124
    10.7.1   Allergic aspergillosis, 124
    10.7.2   Fungus ball of the lung, 125
    10.7.3   Chronic necrotizing aspergillosis of the
          lung, 125
    10.7.4   Acute invasive aspergillosis of the lung, 125
    10.7.5   Tracheobronchitis and obstructing bronchial
          aspergillosis, 128
    10.7.6   Sinusitis, 128
    10.7.7   Cerebral aspergillosis, 129
    10.7.8   Endophthalmitis, 129
    10.7.9   Endocarditis, 129
    10.7.10 Osteomyelitis, 129
    10.7.11 Cutaneous aspergillosis, 130

11   Deep candidosis, 131
11.1 Definition, 131
11.2 Geographical distribution, 131
11.3 The causal organisms and their habitat, 131
11.4 Clinical manifestations, 132
    11.4.1   Oesophagitis, 132
    11.4.2   Gastrointestinal candidosis, 133
    11.4.3   Pulmonary candidosis, 133
    11.4.4   CNS candidosis, 133
    11.4.5   Endocarditis, myocarditis, pericarditis and
          other vascular infections, 134
    11.4.6   Renal candidosis, 135
    11.4.7   Lower urinary tract candidosis, 135
    11.4.8   Peritonitis, 136
    11.4.9   Intrauterine candidosis, 136
    11.4.10 Osteomyelitis, arthritis and myositis, 136
    11.4.11 Endophthalmitis, 137
    11.4.12 Disseminated candidosis, 137
11.5 Candidosis in special hosts, 139
    11.5.1   Low birth-weight infants, 139
    11.5.2   Drug abusers, 139
    11.5.3   Patients with AIDS, 139
11.6 Essential investigations and their interpretation, 140
    11.6.1   Microscopy, 140
    11.6.2   Culture, 140
    11.6.3   Serological tests, 141
11.7 Management, 142
    11.7.1   Oesophagitis, 142
    11.7.2   Meningitis, 143

11.7.3 Endocarditis and vascular infection, 143
11.7.4 Renal candidosis, 144
11.7.5 Lower urinary tract candidosis, 144
11.7.6 Peritonitis, 144
11.7.7 Osteomyelitis and arthritis, 145
11.7.8 Endophthalmitis, 145
11.7.9 Acute disseminated candidosis and candidaemia, 146
11.7.10 Chronic disseminated candidosis, 147

12 Cryptococcosis, 149

12.1 Definition, 149
12.2 Geographical distribution, 149
12.3 The causal organism and its habitat, 149
12.4 Clinical manifestations, 150
    12.4.1 Pulmonary cryptococcosis, 150
    12.4.2 Meningitis, 151
    12.4.3 Cutaneous cryptococcosis, 152
    12.4.4 Osteomyelitis, 152
    12.4.5 Other forms of cryptococcosis, 153
12.5 Cryptococcosis in special hosts, 153
    12.5.1 Patients with AIDS, 153
12.6 Essential investigations and their interpretation, 154
    12.6.1 Microscopy, 154
    12.6.2 Culture, 154
    12.6.3 Serological tests, 154
12.7 Management, 156
    12.7.1 Meningitis and disseminated infection, 156
    12.7.2 Pulmonary cryptococcosis, 158
    12.7.3 Cutaneous cryptococcosis, 159

13 Mucormycosis, 160

13.1 Definition, 160
13.2 Geographical distribution, 160
13.3 The causal organisms and their habitat, 160
13.4 Clinical manifestations, 161
    13.4.1 Rhinocerebral mucormycosis, 161
    13.4.2 Pulmonary mucormycosis, 162
    13.4.3 Gastrointestinal mucormycosis, 162
    13.4.4 Cutaneous mucormycosis, 163
    13.4.5 Disseminated mucormycosis, 163
    13.4.6 Other forms of mucormycosis, 164
13.5 Differential diagnosis, 164
13.6 Essential investigations and their interpretation, 164
    13.6.1 Microscopy, 164
    13.6.2 Culture, 164
    13.6.3 Serological tests, 164

13.7 Management, 165

14 Blastomycosis, 167
14.1 Definition, 167
14.2 Geographical distribution, 167
14.3 The causal organism and its habitat, 167
14.4 Clinical manifestations, 167
    14.4.1 Pulmonary blastomycosis, 168
    14.4.2 Cutaneous blastomycosis, 168
    14.4.3 Osteoarticular blastomycosis, 168
    14.4.4 Genitourinary blastomycosis, 169
    14.4.5 Other forms of disseminated blastomycosis, 169
14.5 Blastomycosis in special hosts, 169
14.6 Differential diagnosis, 170
14.7 Essential investigations and their interpretation, 170
    14.7.1 Microscopy, 170
    14.7.2 Culture, 170
    14.7.3 Serological tests, 171
14.8 Management, 171

15 Coccidioidomycosis, 172
15.1 Definition, 172
15.2 Geographical distribution, 172
15.3 The causal organism and its habitat, 172
15.4 Clinical manifestations, 173
    15.4.1 Primary pulmonary coccidioidomycosis, 173
    15.4.2 Chronic pulmonary coccidioidomycosis, 173
    15.4.3 Disseminated coccidioidomycosis, 174
15.5 Coccidioidomycosis in special hosts, 175
    15.5.1 Patients with AIDS, 175
15.6 Differential diagnosis, 176
15.7 Essential investigations and their interpretation, 176
    15.7.1 Microscopy, 176
    15.7.2 Culture, 177
    15.7.3 Skin tests, 177
    15.7.4 Serological tests, 177
15.8 Management, 178
    15.8.1 Primary pulmonary coccidioidomycosis, 178
    15.8.2 Chronic pulmonary coccidioidomycosis, 179
    15.8.3 Disseminated coccidioidomycosis, 180
    15.8.4 Meningitis, 180

16 Histoplasmosis, 182
16.1 Definition, 182
16.2 Geographical distribution, 182
16.3 The causal organism and its habitat, 182

16.4 Clinical manifestations, 183
 16.4.1 Acute pulmonary histoplasmosis, 183
 16.4.2 Chronic pulmonary histoplasmosis, 184
 16.4.3 Disseminated histoplasmosis, 185
 16.4.4 African histoplasmosis, 186
16.5 Histoplasmosis in special hosts, 186
 16.5.1 Patients with AIDS, 186
16.6 Differential diagnosis, 187
16.7 Essential investigations and their interpretation, 187
 16.7.1 Microscopy, 187
 16.7.2 Culture, 188
 16.7.3 Skin tests, 188
 16.7.4 Serological tests, 188
16.8 Management, 189
 16.8.1 Acute pulmonary histoplasmosis, 189
 16.8.2 Chronic pulmonary histoplasmosis, 189
 16.8.3 Disseminated histoplasmosis, 190

17 Paracoccidioidomycosis, 191
17.1 Definition, 191
17.2 Geographical distribution, 191
17.3 The causal organism and its habitat, 191
17.4 Clinical manifestations, 191
 17.4.1 Chronic pulmonary paracoccidioidomycosis, 192
 17.4.2 Mucocutaneous paracoccidioidomycosis, 192
 17.4.3 Other forms of disseminated paracoccidioidomycosis, 193
17.5 Differential diagnosis, 193
17.6 Essential investigations and their interpretation, 193
 17.6.1 Microscopy, 193
 17.6.2 Culture, 193
 17.6.3 Serological tests, 194
17.7 Management, 194

18 Chromoblastomycosis, 195
18.1 Definition, 195
18.2 Geographical distribution, 195
18.3 The causal organisms and their habitat, 195
18.4 Clinical manifestations, 195
18.5 Differential diagnosis, 196
18.6 Essential investigations and their interpretation, 196
 18.6.1 Microscopy, 196
 18.6.2 Culture, 197
18.7 Management, 197

19 Entomophthoramycoses, 198

19.1 Rhinofacial conidiobolomycosis, 198
    19.1.1 Definition, 198
    19.1.2 Geographical distribution, 198
    19.1.3 The causal organism and its habitat, 198
    19.1.4 Clinical manifestations, 198
    19.1.5 Differential diagnosis, 199
    19.1.6 Essential investigations and their interpretation, 199
    19.1.7 Management, 199
19.2 Basidiobolomycosis, 199
    19.2.1 Definition, 199
    19.2.2 Geographical distribution, 199
    19.2.3 The causal organism and its habitat, 200
    19.2.4 Clinical manifestations, 200
    19.2.5 Differential diagnosis, 200
    19.2.6 Essential investigations and their interpretation, 200
    19.2.7 Management, 200

20 Lobomycosis, 202

20.1 Definition, 202
20.2 Geographical distribution, 202
20.3 The causal organism and its habitat, 202
20.4 Clinical manifestations, 202
20.5 Differential diagnosis, 203
20.6 Essential investigations and their interpretation, 203
    20.6.1 Microscopy, 203
    20.6.2 Culture, 203
20.7 Management, 203

21 Mycetoma, 204

21.1 Definition, 204
21.2 Geographical distribution, 204
21.3 The causal organisms and their habitat, 204
21.4 Clinical manifestations, 205
21.5 Differential diagnosis, 207
21.6 Essential investigations and their interpretation, 207
    21.6.1 Gross examination, 207
    21.6.2 Microscopy, 207
    21.6.3 Culture, 208
21.7 Management, 208

22 Rhinosporidiosis, 210

22.1 Definition, 210
22.2 Geographical distribution, 210
22.3 The causal organism and its habitat, 210

22.4 Clinical manifestations, 210
22.5 Differential diagnosis, 211
22.6 Essential investigations and their interpretation, 211
    22.6.1 Microscopy, 211
    22.6.2 Culture, 211
22.7 Management, 211

23 Sporotrichosis, 212
23.1 Definition, 212
23.2 Geographical distribution, 212
23.3 The causal organism and its habitat, 212
23.4 Clinical manifestations, 212
    23.4.1 Cutaneous sporotrichosis, 213
    23.4.2 Extracutaneous sporotrichosis, 213
23.5 Differential diagnosis, 214
23.6 Essential investigations and their interpretation, 215
    23.6.1 Microscopy, 215
    23.6.2 Culture, 215
    23.6.3 Serological tests, 215
23.7 Management, 215

24 Hyalohyphomycosis, 217
24.1 Definition, 217
24.2 *Fusarium* infection, 217
    24.2.1 Geographical distribution, 217
    24.2.2 The causal organisms and their habitat, 217
    24.2.3 Clinical manifestations, 217
    24.2.4 Essential investigations and their interpretation, 218
    24.2.5 Management, 219
24.3 *Scedosporium* infection, 220
    24.3.1 Geographical distribution, 220
    24.3.2 The causal organisms and their habitat, 220
    24.3.3 Clinical manifestations, 220
    24.3.4 Essential investigations and their interpretation, 221
    24.3.5 Management, 221
24.4 Other agents of hyalohyphomycosis, 222

25 *Penicillium marneffei* infection, 223
25.1 Definition, 223
25.2 Geographical distribution, 223
25.3 The causal organism and its habitat, 223
25.4 Clinical manifestations, 224
25.5 Differential diagnosis, 224
25.6 Essential investigations and their interpretation, 225
    25.6.1 Microscopy, 225

25.6.2   Culture, 225
25.7 Management, 225

26   Phaeohyphomycosis, 227
26.1 Definition, 227
26.2 Geographical distribution, 227
26.3 The causal organisms and their habitat, 227
26.4 Clinical manifestations, 228
    26.4.1   Subcutaneous phaeohyphomycosis, 228
    26.4.2   Paranasal sinus infection, 228
    26.4.3   Cerebral phaeohyphomycosis, 229
    26.4.4   Cutaneous infection, 229
    26.4.5   Other forms of phaeohyphomycosis, 229
26.5 Differential diagnosis, 230
26.6 Essential investigations and their interpretation, 230
    26.6.1   Microscopy, 230
    26.6.2   Culture, 230
26.7 Management, 231
    26.7.1   Subcutaneous phaeohyphomycosis, 231
    26.7.2   Paranasal sinus infection, 231
    26.7.3   Cerebral phaeohyphomycosis, 231
    26.7.4   Cutaneous infection, 231
    26.7.5   Other forms of phaeohyphomycosis, 231

27   Uncommon yeast infections, 232
27.1 Introduction, 232
27.2 Trichosporonosis, 232
    27.2.1   Geographical distribution, 232
    27.2.2   The causal organisms and their habitat, 232
    27.2.3   Clinical manifestations, 232
    27.2.4   Essential investigations and their interpretation, 233
    27.2.5   Management, 234
27.3 Systemic *Malassezia* infection, 234
    27.3.1   Geographical distribution, 234
    27.3.2   The causal organism and its habitat, 235
    27.3.3   Clinical manifestations, 235
    27.3.4   Essential investigations and their interpretation, 235
    27.3.5   Management, 236

Select bibliography, 237

Index, 241

Preface to the second edition

In the 4 years that have elapsed since the first edition of this book was completed there have been a substantial number of significant developments in the diagnosis and management of fungal infections. In particular, new formulations of several antifungal drugs have been introduced and new information about existing agents has become available. As a result clinical management of fungal infections has progressed.

We have tried to include as many of these innovations as possible without, we hope, confusing what is intended to be a concise introduction to the subject. For this second edition, the general format of the book has been retained, but extensive revision has been undertaken and much of the book has been rewritten.

M.D.R., D.W.W.

Preface to the first edition

Fungal infections are assuming a greater importance, largely because of their increasing incidence among transplant patients and other immunocompromised individuals, including those with AIDS. As a result, clinicians and microbiologists alike need to be familiar with the clinical presentation and methods for the diagnosis of these infections, as well as the current treatment choices.

In this book we have attempted to provide a succinct account of the clinical manifestations, laboratory diagnosis and management of fungal infections found in European, American and Australasian practice. The book covers problems encountered both in hospitals and general practice, and is designed to permit clinicians to make the best use of the various laboratory investigations available. Emphasis is placed on clinical presentation, specimen collection, interpretation of laboratory findings, and choice of treatment regimen. In general, the length of the chapters reflects the frequency or the importance of the clinical problem, or both.

We have designed this book to facilitate rapid information retrieval. Our reading list of established literature has been carefully selected to permit efficient access to specific aspects of fungal infections and has been annotated to guide the reader.

We hope this book will be of interest to medical students, junior hospital medical staff, hospital specialists and general practitioners. In particular it should appeal to microbiologists, infectious disease specialists, dermatologists, haematologists, genitourinary medicine specialists, oncologists and intensive-care staff.

M.D.R., D.W.W.

Acknowledgements

We would like to thank our many colleagues, both in the United Kingdom and abroad, whose advice during the various stages of preparation of this edition has been invaluable. As before, especial thanks are due to our wives and families for their tolerance and encouragement.

1   Introduction

The last 20 years have seen unprecedented changes in the pattern of fungal infection in humans. These infections have assumed a much greater importance because of their increasing incidence in patients with the acquired immune deficiency syndrome (AIDS), in transplant recipients, in cancer patients, and in other groups of debilitated or immunocompromised individuals. New pathogens have emerged, while others that once were common have almost been eradicated. Major changes in medical practice, increasing international travel, and misuse of antimicrobial agents, are among the factors that have contributed to this changing pattern of fungal infection. New drugs have been developed, resulting in there now being a choice of treatment depending, to some extent, on the infection and the underlying condition of the patient.

1.1   The nature of fungi

Living organisms are now divided up among no fewer than five Kingdoms, one of which is the Kingdom Fungi. This Kingdom consists of a diverse group of eukaryotic organisms, found throughout nature, that absorb their nourishment from living or dead organic matter.

The classification and identification of fungi is based on their appearance, rather than on the nutritional and biochemical differences that are of such importance in bacterial classification. In moulds, the vegetative stage consists of branching filaments or hyphae, which together form the mycelium. While the hyphae of the more primitive moulds remain aseptate (without cross-walls), those of the more advanced groups are septate, with more or less frequent cross-walls. The individual reproductive bodies of fungi, or spores, consist of a single cell or several cells contained within a rigid wall. During their evolution most fungi have relied upon a combination of sexual and asexual reproductive mechanisms to assist their survival. Their sexual spores and the structures that develop around them form the main basis for fungal classification. In some fungi, however,

1

the asexual stage has proved so successful as a means of rapid dispersal to new habitats, that the sexual stage has diminished or even disappeared. In these fungi the shape of the asexual spores, and the arrangement of the spore-bearing structures are of major importance in identification.

Yeasts are unicellular fungi consisting of separate round, oval or elongated cells that propagate by budding out similar cells from their surface. The bud may become detached from the parent cell, or it may remain attached and itself produce another bud. In this way a chain of cells may be produced. Under certain conditions, continued elongation of the parent cell before it buds results in a chain of elongated cells or pseudohypha. Many fungi, including some of medical importance, can exist in a mycelial or a yeast form depending on the environmental conditions.

1.2 Fungi as human pathogens

Among the 50 000–250 000 species of fungi that have been described, fewer than 200 have been associated with human disease. In general these organisms are free living in nature and are in no way dependent on humans (or animals) for their survival. With few exceptions, fungal infections of humans originate from an exogenous source in the environment and are acquired through inhalation, ingestion or traumatic implantation.

A handful of fungi are capable of causing significant disease in otherwise normal individuals. Many more are only able to produce disease under unusual circumstances, mostly involving host debilitation. However, as a result of the numerous developments in modern medicine, these hitherto innocuous organisms have gained increasing prominence as aetiological agents of disease. Any fungus capable of growing at the temperature of the host (37°C) and surviving in a lowered oxidation-reduction state (a situation found in damaged tissue) must now be regarded as a potential human pathogen.

Fungal infections can be classified into a number of broad groups according to the initial site of infection. Grouping the diseases in this manner brings out clearly the degree of parasitic adaptation of the different groups of fungi and the way in which the site affected is related to the route by which the fungus enters the host.

1.2.1   **The superficial mycoses**
These are infections limited to the outermost layers of the skin, the nails and hair, and the mucous membranes. The principal infections in this group are the dermatophytoses and superficial forms of candidosis. Many of these infections are mild and readily diagnosed, and respond well to treatment.

The dermatophytes are limited to the keratinized tissues of the epidermis, hair and nail. Most are unable to survive as free-living saprotrophs in competition with other keratinophilic organisms in the environment and thus are dependent on passage from host to host for their survival. These obligate pathogens seem to have evolved from unspecialized saprotrophic forms. In the process, most are now no longer capable of sexual reproduction and some are even incapable of asexual reproduction. In general, these organisms have become well adapted to humans, evoking little or no inflammatory reaction from the host.

The aetiological agents of candidosis, like the dermatophytes, are entirely dependent on the living host for their survival, but differ from them in the manner by which this is achieved. These organisms, of which *Candida albicans* is the most important, are normal commensals of the human digestive tract, including the mouth. Acquisition of these organisms from another host seldom results in overt disease, but rather results in the setting-up of a commensal relationship with the new host. These organisms do not produce disease unless some change in the circumstances of the host lowers its natural defences. In this situation, endogenous infection from the host's own reservoir of the organism may result in mucosal, cutaneous or deep-seated infection. In recent years, disseminated candidosis has emerged as a relatively common, life-threatening illness in debilitated or immunocompromised patients.

1.2.2   **The subcutaneous mycoses**
These are infections involving the dermis, subcutaneous tissues and bone. These infections are usually acquired as a result of the traumatic implantation of organisms that grow as saprotrophs in soil and decomposing vegetation. These infections are most frequently encountered among the rural populations of the tropical and subtropical regions of the world, where individuals go barefoot and wear the

minimum of clothing. The disease may remain localized at the site of implantation or spread to adjacent tissue. More widespread dissemination of the infection, through the blood or lymphatics, is uncommon, and usually only occurs if the host is in some way debilitated.

1.2.3   **The systemic mycoses**
These are infections that usually originate in the lungs, but may spread to many other organs. These infections are most commonly acquired as a result of inhaling spores of organisms that grow as saprotrophs in soil or decomposing organic matter, or as pathogens on plants.

The organisms that cause systemic fungal infection can be divided into two distinct groups: the true pathogens and the opportunists. The first of these groups consists of a handful of organisms, such as *Histoplasma capsulatum* and *Coccidioides immitis*, that are able to invade and develop in the tissues of a normal host with no recognizable predisposition. Often these organisms possess unique morphological features that appear to contribute to their survival within the host. The second group, the opportunists, consists of less virulent and less well-adapted organisms, such as *Aspergillus fumigatus*, that are only able to invade the tissues of a debilitated or immunocompromised host.

In most cases, infections with true pathogenic fungi are asymptomatic or mild and of short duration. Many cases occur in regions endemic for the fungus and follow inhalation of spores that have been released into the environment. Individuals who recover from these infections enjoy marked and lasting resistance to reinfection, while the few patients with chronic or residual disease develop a granulomatous response.

In addition to their well-recognized manifestations in normal individuals, infections with true pathogenic fungi have emerged as important diseases in immunocompromised individuals. Histoplasmosis and coccidioidomycosis, for instance, have been recognized as AIDS-defining illnesses. Both diseases are now being seen in significant numbers of patients with AIDS in parts of North and South America. In debilitated or immunocompromised patients, infections with true pathogenic fungi are often life-threatening and unresponsive to antifungal treatment, or relapse following treatment resulting in death.

Opportunistic fungal infections occur in individuals who are debilitated or immunosuppressed as a result of an underlying disease or their treatment. In most cases, infection results in significant disease. Resolution of the infection does not confer protection, and reinfection or reactivation may occur if host resistance is again lowered. Many of the organisms involved are ubiquitous saprotrophs, found in the soil, on decomposing organic matter, and in the air. Although new species of fungi are regularly being identified as causes of disease in immunocompromised patients, four diseases still account for most reported infections: aspergillosis, candidosis, cryptococcosis and mucormycosis (zygomycosis).

Many of the systemic fungal infections of humans have a restricted geographical distribution, being limited to regions where the causal organisms are found in nature. For instance, C. *immitis* only occurs in the soil in certain semi-arid parts of southwestern North America, and similar regions in Central and South America, where there are hot summers and few cold periods in winter. Most cases of human coccidioidomycosis are acquired in these regions. Conversely, *Cryptococcus neoformans* is found wherever there are bird droppings, and cases of cryptococcosis occur throughout the world.

In contrast to the restricted geographical distribution of most of the true pathogenic fungi, the spores of many opportunistic fungi are ubiquitous in the environment and often reach high concentrations in hospital air. Nosocomial (hospital-acquired) outbreaks of aspergillosis and other infections have become associated with hospital construction or renovation work in or near units in which immunosuppressed patients are housed. These outbreaks have highlighted the need for efficient ventilation with filtered air in such units and for careful surveillance.

1.3   **The changing pattern of fungal infection**

Over the past few years, improvements in the management of debilitated medical and surgical patients have led to an unwelcome increase in the number of life-threatening infections due to true pathogenic and opportunistic fungi. These infections are being seen in ever increasing numbers among cancer patients, transplant recipients and patients receiving broad-spectrum antibiotics or parenteral nutrition. Fungal infection is also becoming more common among other groups of debilitated or seriously ill patients, such as drug addicts and patients with AIDS. Estimates of the incidence of these infections are thought to be quite conservative in comparison with their true magnitude, because many fungal infections go undiagnosed.

In addition to the rise in opportunistic fungal infections due to such well-recognized organisms as *A. fumigatus* and *C. albicans*, an ever increasing number of fungi, hitherto regarded as harmless saprotrophs, are being reported as the cause of serious or lethal infection in immunocompromised individuals. For instance, *Trichosporon beigelii*, the aetiological agent of the mild dermatological condition white piedra, is now well documented as a cause of lethal disseminated infection in neutropenic cancer patients and bone marrow transplant recipients. The emergence of this organism as a significant pathogen has important implications for diagnosis and management, because the clinical presentation can mimic candidosis but the organism is often resistant to the drug (amphotericin B) used to treat that infection. The saprotrophic soil mould *Scedosporium apiospermum* is another organism that can cause life-threatening infection that mimics a more common condition, aspergillosis. It, too, is often resistant to amphotericin B, the drug of choice for *Aspergillus* infection.

In certain respects the changing pattern of fungal infection in the developed world is quite different from that seen in the developing world. Throughout the developed world, acquisition of resistance to azole antifungals has become a major issue in patients with AIDS given long-term treatment to suppress persistent oral infection with *C. albicans*. Another significant development has been an apparent rise in the prevalence of species other than *C. albicans* as agents of serious deep-seated *Candida* infection. The precise reasons for this increase are difficult to pinpoint, but changes in medical practice, such as the widespread use of triazole antifungal compounds as prophylactic and therapeutic agents in neutropenic cancer patients and transplant recipients, seem to be important factors in the selection of unusual drug-resistant organisms, such as *Candida glabrata*.

In the developing world, the AIDS epidemic has led to a dramatic increase in the number of deaths from systemic fungal infection, and from histoplasmosis and cryptococcosis in particular. In parts of Africa the incidence of cryptococcosis has risen to more than 30% in patients with AIDS and the number of cases is also increasing in Asia and South America. In parts of South-East Asia the dimorphic mould *Penicillium marneffei* has emerged as the third most common opportunistic infection, after tuberculosis and cryptococcosis. There has also been an unprecedented rise in the number of cases of *P. marneffei* infection diagnosed in European, North American and Australian patients with AIDS, infected during visits to the endemic region.

1.4 Implications for diagnosis and management

The dramatic increase in the number and range of different fungal infections now being reported has been due to a combination of improved recognition and an increasing population of susceptible patients. This rise in prevalence has resulted in an increased awareness of the need for improved methods of diagnosis and for new methods of management. As with other microbial infections, the diagnosis of fungal disease is based upon a combination of clinical observation and laboratory investigation.

Laboratory methods for the diagnosis of fungal infection continue to be updated, but depend for the most part on isolation of the fungus in culture, on its detection in clinical material by direct microscopic examination, and on the detection of an immunological response to the pathogen or some other marker of its presence, such as a metabolic product. Now that an increasing number of common culture contaminants (and other less usual environmental moulds) are occurring as occasional opportunistic pathogens, it is more important than ever that medical microbiologists should be able to recognize these organisms, at least to genus level. The application of molecular biological techniques to the identification of fungi is attracting attention, and while practical procedures have been developed for distinguishing strains of particular organisms, it is doubtful whether these methods can supplant the traditional morphological approach to mould identification.

Molecular biological techniques have also been developed for the detection of fungal pathogens in clinical specimens. In most cases fungal DNA has been detected following amplification by the polymerase chain reaction. Species-specific primers have been designed for a number of organisms, including *A. fumigatus*, *C. albicans* and *C. neoformans*, and several have been used in attempts to detect fungal DNA in specimens, such as blood, urine and cerebrospinal fluid.

Monoclonal antibodies to structural components of the major fungal pathogens of humans are now being produced. These reagents have the potential to form the basis for new tests for identification of organisms. Their introduction has stimulated significant developments in the diagnosis of fungal infection, by enabling improved tests for the detection of circulating fungal antigens in immunocompromised patients to be devised. Monoclonal-based serological tests are now being marketed for the diagnosis of deep candidosis and aspergillosis, as well as for cryptococcosis.

The increased prevalence of life-threatening fungal infection has stimulated interest in the development of new antifungal drugs. New agents, such as the triazoles and the allylamines, have been introduced and new formulations of older compounds, such as lipid-based forms of amphotericin B, have appeared. These developments have improved the treatment of many forms of fungal infection, but problems remain. There are still important infections, such as mucormycosis, for which no reliable treatment has been developed. Then again, many strains of the unusual organisms, such as *Candida krusei* and *T. beigelii*, that are now being isolated from debilitated patients are insensitive to current antifungal compounds.

2   Laboratory diagnosis of fungal infection

2.1   Introduction

As with other microbial infections, the diagnosis of fungal infections depends upon a combination of clinical observation and laboratory investigation. Superficial fungal infections often produce characteristic lesions which suggest a fungal diagnosis, but it is not unusual to find that the appearance of lesions has been modified and rendered atypical by previous treatment. In most situations where deep fungal infection is entertained as a diagnosis, the clinical presentation is non-specific and can be caused by a wide range of infections, underlying illness or complications of treatment. Nor can radiological or other diagnostic imaging methods be relied upon to distinguish fungal infection from other causes of disease.

Laboratory tests can help in establishing or confirming the diagnosis of a fungal infection, in providing objective assessments of response to treatment, and in monitoring resolution of the infection. The successful laboratory diagnosis of fungal infection depends in major part on the collection of appropriate clinical specimens for investigation. It is also dependent on the selection of appropriate microbiological test procedures. These differ from mycosis to mycosis, and depend on the site of infection as well as the presenting symptoms and clinical signs. Interpretation of the results can sometimes be made with confidence, but at times the findings can be unhelpful or even misleading. It is in these situations that close liaison between the clinician and the laboratory is particularly important.

In neutropenic patients and transplant recipients, invasive fungal infection often presents as persistent fever that fails to respond to broad-spectrum antibacterial treatment. The successful management of these patients often depends on the prompt initiation of empirical antifungal treatment without waiting for formal confirmation of the diagnosis. It is essential that these high-risk individuals should be subjected to frequent microbiological surveillance for fungal infection.

2.2 Collection of specimens

To establish or confirm the diagnosis of suspected fungal infection, it is essential for the clinician to provide the laboratory with adequate specimens for investigation. Inappropriate collection, storage or processing of specimens can result in a missed diagnosis. Moreover, to ensure that the most appropriate laboratory tests are performed, it is essential for the clinician to indicate that a fungal infection is suspected and to provide sufficient background information.

In addition to specifying the source of the specimen and its time of collection, it is important to provide information on any underlying illness, recent travel or previous residence abroad, any animal contacts and the patient's occupation if considered relevant. This information will help the laboratory to anticipate which fungal pathogens are most liable to be involved and permit the selection of the most appropriate test procedures. In addition, the laboratory *must* be informed if there are particular risks associated with the handling of the specimen, for instance if the patient has hepatitis or is human immunodeficiency virus (HIV) positive.

With the exception of skin, hair and nails, specimens for mycological examination should be collected into and transported to the laboratory in sterile containers appropriate to the type of material being investigated. All specimen containers should be clearly labelled.

2.2.1 Skin, nails and hair

Skin, nails and hair should be collected into folded squares of black paper (about 10 × 10 cm). The use of paper permits the specimen to dry out, which helps to reduce bacterial contamination and also provides a convenient means of storing specimens for long periods (12 months or longer). It is often helpful to clean superficial lesions with 70% alcohol prior to sampling as this will improve the chances of detecting fungus on microscopic examination, as well as reducing the likelihood of bacterial contamination of cultures. Prior cleaning is essential if ointments, creams or powders have been applied to the lesion.

Material should be collected from cutaneous lesions by scraping outwards from the margin of the lesion with a blunt scalpel. If there is minimal scaling, it is helpful to use

clear adhesive tape, or adhesive skin sampling discs, to remove material for examination. The sellotape strip or disc should be pressed against the lesion, peeled off and placed, adhesive side down, on a clean glass microscope slide for transportation to the laboratory.

It is often helpful to use a Wood's light to select infected scalp hairs for laboratory investigation. If none of the hairs give the green fluorescence which is a feature of some forms of dermatophyte scalp infection, a search should be made for lustreless hairs or stumps, and for hairs broken off at follicle mouths. Hairs should be plucked from the scalp with forceps. Cut hairs without roots are unsuitable for mycological investigation because the infection is usually confined near or below the surface of the scalp.

Another method which is useful for collection of adequate material from patients with inconspicuous scalp lesions is to brush the scalp with a plastic massage pad which is then pressed into the surface of an agar plate. The pad should be sterilized in 1% chlorhexidine for 1 h and rinsed in sterile water before being reused.

Nail specimens should be taken from any discoloured, dystrophic or brittle parts of the nail. Specimens should be cut as far back as possible from the edge of the nail and should include the full thickness of the nail because some fungi are confined to the lower parts. If the nail is thickened, scrapings can also be taken from beneath it.

2.2.2 Mucous membranes

Although scrapings from oral lesions are better than swabs for diagnosis of oral infections, the latter are more frequently used, mainly because they are more convenient for transporting material to the laboratory. Swabs should either be moistened with sterile water or saline prior to taking the sample, or sent to the laboratory in transport medium.

For vaginal infections, swabs should be taken from discharge in the vagina and from the lateral vaginal wall. Swabs should be sent to the laboratory in transport medium.

2.2.3 Ear

Scrapings of material from the ear canal are to be preferred, although swabs can also be used.

2.2.4 **Eye**

Material from a corneal ulcer with a suspected fungal cause should be collected by scraping the ulcer with a sterile platinum spatula. The entire base of the ulcer as well as the edges should be sampled. Because the amount of material that can be obtained will be small, it is best transferred to an agar plate for culture and to a glass slide for microscopic examination at the bedside. The plate should be marked to indicate the point of inoculation before being sent to the laboratory. Swabs are not suitable for sampling corneal lesions.

In patients with suspected fungal endophthalmitis, vitreous humour should be collected whenever possible. Vitreous humour specimens that have been diluted by the irrigating solution should be concentrated by centrifugation before being examined in the laboratory.

2.2.5 **Blood**

Blood culture should be performed in all cases of suspected deep fungal infection. However, unless specialized techniques or media are used, clinicians should not expect blood cultures taken for isolation of bacteria to detect fungi other than *Candida* species, *Cryptococcus neoformans*, or *Trichosporon* species. Isolation of fungi from blood depends on a number of factors, including the amount of blood sampled, the number of samples collected, and the method of processing. Culture of arterial blood should be considered if venous blood cultures are unsuccessful in a patient with suspected deep mycosis.

The best fungal blood culture method appears to be the Isolator lysis centrifugation system (DuPont), both in terms of the isolation rate and the time taken to recover the organisms. The best results with this system have been reported from North American hospitals, due in major part to the increased isolation rate of *Histoplasma capsulatum* and, to a lesser extent, *C. neoformans*. Elsewhere, it is often impracticable to use this expensive and labour-intensive method of blood culture on a routine basis. Good results have also been obtained with several other commercial systems, including the Septi-Chek biphasic system (Becton-Dickenson) and the high-volume resin medium provided for the non-radiometric Bactec system (Becton-Dickenson).

Isolation of fungi from blood cultures can be improved in several ways. First, by employing more than one method. This can be achieved by adding an Isolator tube or the Bactec fungal medium to the standard set for selected patients. Second, by ensuring that an adequate amount of blood is cultured (at least 20 ml). Third, by ensuring that blood cultures from high-risk patients are subcultured and incubated for a further 2 weeks.

2.2.6 Cerebrospinal fluid

Cerebrospinal fluid (CSF) specimens of 3–5 ml are ideal, but are often smaller than this. Samples can be centrifuged and the supernatant fluid used for serological tests. The sediment can be cultured, but is also useful for microscopic examination.

2.2.7 Urine

In non-catheterized patients, fresh mid-stream specimens of urine are adequate for mycological investigation, provided care is taken to ensure that vaginal or perineal infection does not lead to contamination. In infants, suprapubic aspiration is the best method of urine collection. Urine samples should be processed for microscopic examination and culture, but can also be tested for fungal antigens.

Patients with blastomycosis or cryptococcosis may have prostatic infection, and it is therefore important to collect urine specimens following prostatic massage. The specimen should be centrifuged and the sediment cultured. Other disseminated infections that can be diagnosed on the basis of a positive urine culture include coccidioidomycosis and histoplasmosis.

2.2.8 Other fluids

Chest, abdominal and joint fluids, whether aspirated or drained, should be collected into sterile containers which include a small amount of sterile heparin (diluted 1 : 1000) to prevent clotting. The specimens should be centrifuged and the sediment cultured. Drain fluid from patients on continuous peritoneal dialysis should be collected in a sterile container without heparin.

2.2.9 Lower respiratory tract specimens

Fresh, early morning samples of sputum are ideal. These

should be collected in sterile containers and processed within 2 h of collection. If delay in processing is unavoidable, specimens must be stored at 4°C. If the patient does not have a productive cough, a sputum sample may be induced by introducing nebulized saline into the bronchial tree. It is recommended that at least three samples of sputum be submitted for microscopic examination and culture whenever a fungal infection is suspected: 24-h collections of sputum are not suitable for mycological investigation.

In immunocompromised patients, the most useful procedures for collection of lower respiratory tract specimens are bronchoalveolar lavage or a bronchial wash. These procedures are carried out with a fibre-optic bronchoscope and provide good material for microscopic examination and culture. Specimens should be centrifuged and the sediment examined.

Percutaneous needle biopsies are useful in patients with focal lung disease, in particular those with peripheral lesions which are not accessible to a bronchoscope. Large needles are better than fine needles and the procedure should be carried out under radiological guidance. Specimens should be processed for microscopic examination and culture.

2.2.10 Pus

If possible, swabs should not be used to collect material from draining abscesses or ulcers. If a swab must be used, then material should be taken from as deep as possible within the lesion. Pus from undrained subcutaneous abscesses or sinus tracts should be aspirated with a sterile needle and syringe. If grains are visible in the pus (as in mycetoma), these should be collected. In mycetoma, if the crusts at the opening of sinus tracts are lifted, grains can often be found in the pus underneath.

2.2.11 Bone marrow

These specimens are useful for making the diagnosis in a number of deep fungal infections, including histoplasmosis, cryptococcosis and paracoccidioidomycosis. About 3–5 ml aspirated material should be collected into a sterile container which includes a small amount of sterile heparin (diluted 1:1000).

2.2.12 Tissue

Tissue specimens should be placed in sterile saline and *not* in formalin. If possible, material should be obtained from both the middle and the edge of lesions. Total excision of small cutaneous, subcutaneous or mucosal lesions is often possible.

2.3 **Specimens for serological tests**

Serological tests for fungal pathogens are often more helpful if paired or sequential specimens are collected. Blood, CSF, urine and other biological fluids for serological testing should be collected into glass or plastic tubes without anticoagulants; 5–10 ml is usually sufficient.

2.4 **Specimens for antifungal drug level determinations**

The concentrations of antifungal drugs are measured for two principal reasons: (i) to ensure that adequate drug concentrations are attained; and (ii) to ensure that concentrations that could cause unpleasant or even harmful side-effects are avoided.

Blood and other biological fluids should be collected into glass or plastic tubes without anticoagulants; 5–10 ml is usually sufficient. Care should be taken to ensure that specimens are taken at the most appropriate times: samples should be collected just before a dose is due and/or around the expected time of peak blood concentrations (see Chapter 3).

2.5 **Transport of specimens**

Apart from specimens from cases of suspected dermatophytosis which can often be stored for weeks or even months before processing, specimens for mycological investigation must be processed as soon as possible after collection. Delay may result in the death of fastidious organisms, in overgrowth of contaminants, and/or multiplication in the number of organisms present.

Specimens mailed to laboratories must be packaged and labelled according to the guidelines laid down for the transport of biological material by the relevant postal authorities. Metal canisters are now recommended for packaging of certain hazardous materials, such as specimens from HIV-positive individuals. Plastic petri dishes are unsuitable for sending through the mail. The specimen container or culture should be sealed within a plastic bag before packaging, so that any breakage and subsequent spillage is contained. The sender's name should be clearly marked on the outside of the package so that they may be contacted for instructions should a problem arise.

2.6 Interpretation of laboratory test results

Interpretation of the results of laboratory tests can sometimes be made with confidence, but at times the findings may be unhelpful or even misleading. The investigations available include microscopic examination, culture and serological tests. The choice of appropriate tests differs from mycosis to mycosis, and depends on the site of infection as well as the presenting symptoms and clinical signs. It must always be appreciated that every laboratory test has its limitations, and that negative results can be obtained which may lead to unjustified exclusion of a mycological diagnosis.

2.6.1 Direct microscopic examination

The direct microscopic examination of clinical material is one of the simpler and most helpful procedures for the laboratory diagnosis of fungal infection. Various methods can be used: unstained wet-mount preparations may be examined by light-field, dark-field or phase-contrast illumination; or dried smears can be stained and examined. Chemical brighteners, such as calcofluor white, can be helpful in revealing fungal elements in wet mounts of sputum, skin and other clinical materials when examined under a fluorescence microscope.

Direct microscopic examination is most useful in the diagnosis of superficial and subcutaneous fungal infections. Recognition of fungal elements in skin scrapings, hair or nail specimens can provide a reliable indication of the mycosis involved, whether it be dermatophytosis, candidosis or pityriasis versicolor. In certain situations, direct microscopic examination of fluids or other clinical material can establish the diagnosis of a deep mycosis. Instances include the detection of encapsulated *C. neoformans* cells in CSF, or *H. capsulatum* cells in peripheral blood smears. More often, however, only a tentative diagnosis of deep fungal infection can be made on the basis of microscopic examination. Nevertheless, this is often sufficient to allow the instigation of antifungal treatment pending the outcome of other investigations.

2.6.2 **Culture**

With few exceptions the isolation of pathogenic fungi from clinical material is not difficult. Should the isolate be identified as an unequivocal pathogen, such as *Trichophyton rubrum* or *C. neoformans*, then the diagnosis is established. If, however, an opportunistic pathogen such as *Aspergillus fumigatus* or *Candida albicans* is recovered, then its isolation may have no clinical relevance unless there is additional evidence of infection. Isolation of opportunistic fungal pathogens from sterile sites, such as blood or CSF, often provides reliable evidence of significant infection, but their isolation from material such as pus, sputum or urine must be interpreted with caution. Attention should be given to the amount of fungus isolated and further investigations undertaken.

Many unfamiliar organisms have been reported to cause deep-seated fungal infection in immunocompromised patients. No isolate should be dismissed as a contaminant without careful consideration of the clinical condition of the patient, the site of isolation, the method of specimen collection and the amount of organisms recovered.

Although culture often provides the definitive diagnosis of a fungal infection, it also has some limitations. Chief amongst these is failure to recover the organism. This may be due to inadequate specimen collection or delayed transport of specimens. Incorrect isolation procedures or inadequate periods of incubation are other important factors. It is essential for the clinician to inform the laboratory if a particular fungal infection is suspected and provide sufficient information to permit the most appropriate culture procedures to be followed.

The isolation and identification of a mycelial fungus can take several weeks. In such unavoidable instances, the result may become available too late either to help with the diagnosis or with the choice of treatment. Nevertheless, culture should always be attempted so that a definitive diagnosis can be obtained. One recent development that has shortened the length of time required for identification of some dimorphic fungal pathogens has been the introduction of commercial DNA probes (Gen-Probe) for *H. capsulatum*, *Coccidioides immitis* and *Blastomyces dermatitidis*.

2.6.3   **Serological tests**

The detection of fungal antibodies is sometimes helpful in the diagnosis of subcutaneous and deep-seated fungal infections. Numerous methods are available. For some infections, such as histoplasmosis and coccidioidomycosis, the tests are reliable, but for others the results are seldom more than suggestive or supportive of a fungal diagnosis. It is often more helpful if sequential tests can be performed, so that rising levels of antibodies may be detected.

Tests for the detection of fungal antibodies are least helpful in immunocompromised patients. In such cases serological tests for the detection of fungal antigens may be more useful. Antigen detection is an established procedure for the diagnosis of cryptococcosis and similar methods have been introduced for other mycoses, including aspergillosis, candidosis and histoplasmosis. Because of the low concentrations of circulating antigens present in many infected individuals, sensitive test methods are required. Negative results do not, however, exclude the diagnosis.

2.6.4   **Histopathological examination**

The demonstration of fungal elements in histological material is one of the most useful procedures for the diagnosis of subcutaneous and deep-seated fungal infections. The ease with which a fungal pathogen can be recognized in tissue is dependent in part on its abundance, but also on the distinctiveness of its appearance. Although there are a number of special stains for detecting and highlighting fungal cells, specific identification of organisms may be difficult. The detection of non-pigmented, branching, septate mycelium can be indicative of *Aspergillus* infection, but it is also characteristic of a number of less common organisms. Likewise, the detection of small budding cells in clinical material seldom permits a specific diagnosis. Tissue-form cells of *H. capsulatum* and *B. dermatitidis*, for instance, can appear similar and may be confused with non-encapsulated *C. neoformans* cells.

Immunofluorescence and other immunochemical staining procedures sometimes permit the specific identification of fungal elements in histopathological sections. These methods have been applied to the diagnosis of a number of mycotic infections, including aspergillosis, candidosis and mucormycosis. Immunochemical staining can facilitate the identification of atypical fungal elements and the detection of small numbers of organisms. It can also assist with the diagnosis of mixed infections.

3   Antifungal drugs

3.1   Introduction

In comparison with the number of antibacterial drugs available, there are far fewer antifungal compounds. Even so the number of antifungal drugs is increasing all the time. There are three major families of compounds: the polyenes, azoles and allylamines. In addition there is a miscellaneous group of compounds, such as griseofulvin, which do not belong to one of the major families. This is not a static picture and there are new groups of compounds under development all the time.

This chapter reviews the principal antifungals in current use for superficial, subcutaneous and deep-seated fungal infections.

3.2   Amphotericin B

Amphotericin B is a macrocyclic polyene antibiotic derived from *Streptomyces nodosus*. It remains the drug of choice for many forms of deep fungal infection.

Parenteral administration of the conventional micellar suspension formulation of amphotericin B is often associated with unpleasant infusion-related reactions and treatment-limiting toxic effects, in particular renal impairment. This problem has led to the development of three lipid-based formulations of the drug: (i) liposomal amphotericin B (AmBisome) in which the drug is encapsulated in phospholipid-containing liposomes; (ii) amphotericin B lipid complex (Abelcet, ABLC) in which it is complexed with phospholipids to form ribbon-like structures; and (iii) amphotericin B colloidal dispersion (Amphocil, Amphotec, ABCD) in which the drug is complexed with cholesterol sulphate to form small lipid discs. These formulations appear to be less toxic than the micellar suspension because of their altered pharmacological distribution.

3.2.1   Mechanism of action

Amphotericin B binds to ergosterol, the principal sterol in the membrane of susceptible fungal cells, causing impairment of membrane barrier function, loss of cell constituents, metabolic disruption and cell death. In addition to its membrane permeabilizing effects, the drug can cause oxidative damage to fungal cells. Mammalian cell membranes also contain sterols and it has been suggested that amphotericin B-induced damage to human and fungal cells shares common mechanisms.

3.2.2   **Spectrum of action**
Amphotericin B has a broad spectrum of action including *Aspergillus fumigatus*, *Blastomyces dermatitidis*, *Candida* species, *Coccidioides immitis*, *Cryptococcus neoformans*, *Histoplasma capsulatum*, and *Paracoccidioides brasiliensis*. *Fusarium* species and some other *Aspergillus* species may be less susceptible, while *Scedosporium* species and *Trichosporon* species may be resistant.

3.2.3   **Acquired resistance**
Treatment failure attributable to the development of amphotericin B resistance is rare. Resistant strains of *Candida lusitaniae* and *C. tropicalis*, with qualitative and quantitative alterations in membrane sterol composition, including reduced amounts of ergosterol, have been isolated during treatment. Resistant strains of *C. neoformans* have been isolated from a few patients with the acquired immune deficiency syndrome (AIDS) with relapsing cryptococcosis, but this is an uncommon problem at present.

3.2.4   **Pharmacokinetics**
Amphotericin B is not absorbed following mucosal or cutaneous application. Minimal absorption occurs from the gastrointestinal tract. Oral administration of a 3-g dose will produce serum concentrations in the region of 0.1–0.5 mg/l.

CONVENTIONAL FORMULATION
Parenteral administration of a 1 mg/kg dose of the conventional formulation of the drug will produce maximum serum concentrations of 1.0–2.0 mg/l. Less than 10% of the dose remains in the blood 12 h after administration and more than 90% of this is protein-bound. Most of the remainder can be found in the liver (up to 40% of the dose), lungs (up to 6%), and kidneys (up to 2%). Levels in cerebrospinal fluid (CSF) are less than 5% of the simultaneous

blood concentration. Amphotericin B binds to tissues for prolonged periods of time, re-entering the circulation slowly from these storage sites. The conventional formulation has a second-phase elimination half-life of about 24–48 h and a third-phase half-life of about 2 weeks.

LIPID-BASED FORMULATIONS

The pharmacokinetics of the different lipid-based formulations of amphotericin B are quite diverse. Large structures, such as ABLC, are rapidly removed from the blood, but smaller liposomes remain in the circulation for much longer periods.

The maximum serum concentrations obtained after parenteral administration of liposomal amphotericin B (AmBisome) have ranged from 10 to 35 mg/l for a 3 mg/kg dose and from 25 to 60 mg/l for a 5 mg/kg dose. Levels of 5–10 mg/l have been detected 24 h after a 5 mg/kg dose. In animals, administration of liposomal amphotericin B results in much higher drug concentrations in the liver and spleen than are achieved with conventional amphotericin B. Levels in renal tissue are much lower than those obtained with equivalent amounts of the conventional formulation. Human tissue distribution has not been studied in detail, but the highest drug levels occur in the liver and spleen.

The maximum serum concentrations obtained after parenteral administration of ABLC are lower than after administration of equivalent amounts of conventional amphotericin B due to more rapid distribution of the drug to tissue. Maximum levels have ranged from 1 to 2 mg/l for a 5 mg/kg dose. In animals, administration of ABLC results in much higher drug concentrations in the liver, spleen and lungs than are achieved with conventional amphotericin B. Levels in renal tissue are much lower than those obtained with equivalent amounts of the conventional formulation. Human tissue distribution has not been studied in detail.

Maximum serum concentrations of about 2 mg/l have been obtained following a 1 mg/kg dose of ABCD, but levels in the blood decline soon after the end of the infusion due to rapid distribution of the drug to tissue. In animals, administration of ABCD results in much higher drug concentrations in the liver and spleen than are achieved with conventional amphotericin B. Levels in renal tissue are much lower than those obtained with equivalent amounts of the conventional formulation. Human tissue distribution has not been studied in detail.

3.2.5 Metabolism

No metabolites have been identified, but it is thought that amphotericin B is metabolized in the liver. Less than 5% of a given dose is excreted unchanged in the urine. Blood concentrations are unchanged in hepatic or renal failure. Likewise, haemodialysis does not reduce blood levels unless the patient is hyperlipaemic in which case there is some drug loss due to adherence to the dialysis membrane.

3.2.6 Pharmaceutics

Amphotericin B is available in oral, topical and parenteral forms.

CONVENTIONAL FORMULATION

Amphotericin B is supplied for parenteral administration in lyophilized form in 50-mg amounts together with 41 mg sodium deoxycholate (which acts as a dispersing agent) and a sodium phosphate buffer. The addition of 10 ml sterile water gives a clear micellar suspension. This is further diluted with 490 ml 5% dextrose solution prior to injection to give a final drug concentration of 100 mg/l. The dextrose solution should have a pH of 4.2 or greater to prevent precipitation of the drug. The diluted drug should be used within 24 h, but does not need to be protected from light. Other preparations for injection should not be added to an amphotericin B infusion. If there are signs of precipitation, the infusion must be discarded.

LIPID-BASED FORMULATIONS

Liposomal amphotericin B (AmBisome) is supplied for parenteral administration in lyophilized form in 50-mg amounts and is first reconstituted in 12 ml sterile water (for injection) to give a drug concentration of 4 mg/ml. The drug solution is further diluted with between one and 19 parts of 5% dextrose (for injection) to give a final drug concentration in the range of 0.2–2.0 mg/ml amphotericin B and filter sterilized. The reconstituted drug in water can be stored in a refrigerator for up to 24 h prior to dilution with 5% dextrose solution. Infusion of the drug should be commenced within 6 h of dilution with 5% dextrose solution.

ABLC is supplied for parenteral administration as a sterile suspension in 100-mg amounts which must be filter sterilized and diluted before use with 5% dextrose (for injection) to a final infusion volume of about 500 ml (250 ml in children). The diluted suspension can be stored in a refrigerator for up to 15 h prior to infusion.

ABCD is supplied for parenteral administration in lyophilized form in 50- or 100-mg amounts and is first reconstituted in 10 or 20 ml sterile water (for injection) to give a drug concentration of 5 mg/ml. The drug solution is then diluted eightfold with 5% dextrose (for injection) to give a final concentration of 0.625 mg/ml amphotericin B. The reconstituted drug in water can be stored in a refrigerator for up to 24 h prior to dilution with 5% dextrose solution. After further dilution with 5% dextrose solution, the drug should be stored in a refrigerator and used within 24 h.

To avoid precipitation, liposomal amphotericin B, ABLC and ABCD must not be reconstituted or diluted with saline and should not be mixed with other drugs. Existing lines must be flushed with 5% dextrose solution prior to the infusion or, if this is not feasible, a separate line should be used.

3.2.7 Therapeutic use

Topical amphotericin B preparations can be used to treat mucosal and cutaneous forms of candidosis.

Parenteral amphotericin B is still the drug of choice for many forms of deep fungal infection, including blastomycosis, coccidioidomycosis, cryptococcosis, histoplasmosis and paracoccidioidomycosis. It is also effective in certain forms of mucormycosis, hyalohyphomycosis and phaeohyphomycosis. However, it is often ineffective in *Scedosporium* infection and trichosporonosis, as well as in aspergillosis and candidosis in neutropenic patients. Administration of the conventional formulation of the drug is associated with harmful side-effects and unpleasant reactions which often limit the amount that can be given.

Lipid-based formulations of amphotericin B are better tolerated and higher doses can be given over shorter periods with fewer toxic reactions. These formulations are indicated for the treatment of serious infections in patients who have failed to respond to conventional amphotericin B, or who have developed severe side-effects to conventional amphotericin B, or in whom conventional amphotericin B is contraindicated because of renal impairment.

The conventional parenteral formulation of amphotericin B has been instilled into a number of sites, including the bladder, peritoneum and joints. However, intraperitoneal infusion of the drug is painful and has been associated with adhesion formation.

3.2.8   **Mode of administration**
The dose and duration of topical treatment will differ from patient to patient and depend on the nature and extent of infection. The usual adult dose of the oral suspension for oral forms of candidosis is 1–2 ml (100–200 mg) at 6-h intervals. As the drug is not absorbed the success of treatment depends on maintaining an adequate concentration in the mouth for as long as possible. The recommended dosage of the oral suspension for infants and children is 1 ml (100 mg) at 6-h intervals.

CONVENTIONAL FORMULATION
Most patients with deep fungal infection are treated with 1–2 g amphotericin B over 6–10 weeks, but this will differ from person to person, depending upon the nature and extent of the infection and the underlying illness. In adults with normal renal function the usual dose is between 0.5 and 1.0 mg/kg. For empirical treatment the dose should be 1.0 mg/kg. There is no evidence to support the clinical prejudice that a lower dose can be used in suspected candidosis.

An initial test dose of 1 mg amphotericin B in 50 ml dextrose solution should be given over 1–2 h (0.5 mg in children weighing less than 30 kg), with general clinical observation and monitoring of temperature, pulse and blood pressure at 30-min intervals. This is because occasional patients have an idiosyncratic reaction of severe hypotension or an anaphylaxis-like reaction. In the few patients with a reaction, the test infusion should be discontinued, supportive treatment including hydrocortisone should be given, and a repeat test dose administered over a longer period. If the test dose is well tolerated, there can be progression to larger doses. Several dosage regimens are available (see Tables 3.1 and 3.2).

In patients who are not immunocompromised or suffering a serious life-threatening infection, optimum dosage is best

Table 3.1 Regimens for rapid escalation of amphotericin B dosage.

Time infusion started (h)	Duration of infusion (h)	Dosage (mg)	Volume of solution 1 (ml)	Volume of solution 2 (ml)
0	2	1	10	40
4	6	24	240	760
16	6	25	250	750
40	6	50	500	500

(then at 24-h intervals; dose not to exceed 50 mg or 1.0 mg/kg per infusion whichever is the lesser)

0	2	1	10	40
2	6	9	90	360
12	6	10	100	400
24	6	20	200	300
48	6	30	300	700
72	6	40	400	600
96	6	50	500	500

(then at 24-h intervals; dose not to exceed 50 mg or 1.0 mg/kg per infusion whichever is the lesser)

Solution 1: amphotericin B at 100 mg/l in 5% dextrose solution.
Solution 2: 5% dextrose solution.

Table 3.2 Regimen for gradual escalation of amphotericin B dosage.

Time infusion started (h)	Duration of infusion (h)	Dosage (mg)	Volume of solution 1 (ml)	Volume of solution 2 (ml)
0	2	1	10	40
2	6	9	90	360
24	6	10	100	400
48	6	20	200	300
72	6	30	300	700
96	6	40	400	600
120	6	50	500	500

(then at 24-h intervals; dose not to exceed 50 mg or 1.0 mg/kg per infusion whichever is the lesser)

Solution 1: amphotericin B at 100 mg/l in 5% dextrose solution.
Solution 2: 5% dextrose solution.

achieved through gradual augmentation of the dose. The dose can be increased up to 1.0 mg/kg, but individual infusions should not contain more than 50 mg of the drug.

In immunosuppressed patients and others with a serious infection, the dose of amphotericin B should be increased as rapidly as the patient's tolerance of the drug will allow. Rapid augmentation of the dose carries a greater risk of acute renal failure, but immunosuppressed patients often tolerate these regimens well.

Four-hour infusions appear to be as well tolerated as the more traditional 6-h infusion period in patients with normal renal function. However, it is not advisable to give the infusion over less than 4 h.

After 2 weeks of treatment, blood concentrations become stable, tissue levels begin to accumulate and it becomes possible to administer the drug at 48- or 72-h intervals. The maximum dose can then be increased from 1.0 to 1.5 mg/kg.

Intrathecal administration of amphotericin B is often associated with side-effects and complications, and oral triazole treatment has largely replaced this form of management in patients with fungal meningitis. Intracisternal injection is to be preferred to lumbar intrathecal administration, because of the risk of chronic lumbar arachnoiditis, but even with this the meninges become damaged and a subcutaneous reservoir may be required to deliver the drug to the CSF. Injections should be given two or three times per week, with the dose increased from 0.025 mg as tolerated to 0.25–1.0 mg.

Lower urinary tract candidosis will often respond to local treatment with amphotericin B (see Chapter 11). Both continuous irrigation (50 mg/l in sterile water) and intermittent instillation (200–300 ml of a 50 mg/l solution at 6–8-h intervals) for 5–7 days have been used.

LIPID-BASED FORMULATIONS

It is not possible to define the total dosage requirements and duration of treatment needed to cure particular fungal infections. For this reason, the dosage of lipid-based formulations of amphotericin B should be adjusted to the individual requirements of each patient. It is prudent to give an initial test dose of 1 mg to all patients (0.5 mg in children weighing less than 30 kg) because of the risk of anaphylactoid reactions.

It is usual to begin treatment with liposomal amphotericin B (AmBisome) with a dose of 1.0 mg/kg, but this can be increased to 3.0 mg/kg or even higher. This formulation is infused over a 30–60-min period. Liposomal amphotericin B has been administered to individual patients for up to 3 months, to a cumulative dosage of 15 g without significant toxic side-effects. However, a cumulative dosage of 1–3 g given over 3–4 weeks has been more typical.

The recommended dosage of ABLC is 5 mg/kg and this should be infused over a 2-h period for at least 2 weeks. This formulation of amphotericin B has been administered to individual patients for up to 11 months, to a cumulative dosage of 50 g without significant toxic side-effects.

It is usual to begin treatment with ABCD with a dose of 1.0 mg/kg, increasing to the recommended dose of 3.0–4.0 mg/kg as required. This formulation is infused over a 60–90-min period. ABCD has been administered to individual patients to a cumulative dosage of 3 g without significant toxic side-effects.

3.2.9 Adverse reactions

CONVENTIONAL FORMULATION

The immediate side-effects of the intravenous infusion of amphotericin B include fever, chills and rigors. These unpleasant reactions differ from patient to patient, but usually begin 1–3 h after starting the infusion and last for about an hour. They are most common during the first week of treatment and often diminish thereafter. These reactions can be prevented or reduced by either slowing the rate of infusion or by giving 25 mg of parenteral hydrocortisone just before the infusion is started or 25–50 mg during it if a reaction occurs. Parenteral chlorpheniramine (12.5–25 mg) or oral ibuprofen (10 mg/kg) can also reduce chills if given prior to the infusion.

Nausea and vomiting occur less frequently and, just as with fever and rigors, often diminish as treatment proceeds. Premedication with antiemetics is helpful.

Local phlebitis from intravenous administration of the conventional formulation of amphotericin B is common. If the drug is given through a peripheral vein, the infusion site should be changed for each dose. Phlebitis can be prevented or ameliorated by slowing the rate of the infusion or by adding a small amount of heparin (500–1000 units/l) to the solution.

The most serious toxic effect of amphotericin B is renal tubular damage. Most patients receiving the conventional formulation of the drug suffer some impairment of renal function, but it occurs most often in individuals given more than 0.5 mg/kg per day. Infants and children are less susceptible to the nephrotoxic effects of amphotericin B. Renal function will return to almost normal levels in most patients several months after treatment has ceased, but irreversible renal failure can occur.

Renal damage can be reduced or prevented by careful monitoring during treatment. In the stable patient, renal function should be measured twice weekly and the treatment interrupted or the dosage modified if the serum creatinine concentration exceeds 250 μmol/l. Intravenous sodium supplementation may help to prevent amphotericin B-induced renal impairment.

Amphotericin B also causes renal wasting of potassium and magnesium due to renal tubular damage and this can reach symptomatic proportions. Serum concentrations of potassium and magnesium should be monitored at regular intervals. Their loss can be reduced by administering 10–20 mg of oral amiloride per day, but intravenous electrolyte supplements must be given if low levels are seen.

Patients treated for more than 2 weeks often develop a mild normochromic, normocytic anaemia. Blood transfusion may be of benefit, but is not usually required.

Pulmonary reactions, with acute dyspnoea, hypoxaemia and interstitial infiltrates, can occur when treatment with amphotericin B is combined with granulocyte transfusion. For this reason it is advisable to separate the infusion of the drug from the time of granulocyte transfusion.

LIPID-BASED FORMULATIONS

The prevalence of immediate side-effects after administration of ABLC or ABCD is lower than reported for conventional amphotericin B. Fever and chills are the most common adverse effects of these formulations. These side-effects tend to occur during the first few days of treatment, but respond to premedication with hydrocortisone. Immediate toxic reactions are rare during liposomal amphotericin B (AmBisome) treatment.

Renal impairment is uncommon in patients treated with lipid-based formulations of amphotericin B. Moreover, individuals who develop renal impairment during treatment with the conventional formulation can be stabilized or improved when lipid-based amphotericin B is substituted, even when the dose is increased. Renal function should be monitored at regular intervals, particularly in patients receiving other nephrotoxic drugs.

3.2.10 **Drug interactions**

Amphotericin B can augment the nephrotoxic effects of other drugs, such as aminoglycoside antibiotics, cyclosporin and certain antineoplastic agents. These drugs should be administered together with caution. Amphotericin B can also augment corticosteroid-induced potassium loss and the resulting hypokalaemia may enhance the action of digitalis glycosides.

Amphotericin B and flucytosine have an additive or synergistic effect when used in combination against *Candida* species or *C. neoformans*.

3.3 **Fluconazole**

Fluconazole is a synthetic bis-triazole compound.

3.3.1 **Mechanism of action**

Fluconazole is a potent inhibitor of ergosterol biosynthesis, through its action on the cytochrome P-450-dependent enzyme, lanosterol 14α-demethylase. Depletion of ergosterol, the principal sterol in the membrane of susceptible fungal cells, and accumulation of methylated sterols leads to alterations in a number of membrane-associated cell functions.

3.3.2 **Spectrum of action**

Fluconazole has a broad spectrum of action including *Blastomyces dermatitidis*, *Coccidioides immitis*, *Cryptococcus neoformans*, *Histoplasma capsulatum* and *Paracoccidioides brasiliensis*. It is active against *Candida albicans*, *C. tropicalis* and *C. parapsilosis*, but many strains of *C. krusei* and *Torulopsis glabrata* (now reclassified as *Candida glabrata*) appear to be insensitive. Fluconazole is active in dermatophytosis, but appears to be ineffective in aspergillosis and mucormycosis.

In neutropenic patients, the most common manifestation of fluconazole resistance is the selection of unusual *Candida* species, such as *C. krusei*, which possess intrinsic resistance to the drug.

3.3.3 Acquired resistance

There have been few reports of resistance developing in *C. albicans* or *C. tropicalis* during short-term fluconazole treatment in patients with mucosal or deep-seated forms of candidosis. In patients with AIDS, resistant strains of *C. albicans* often appear as a result of repeated courses of low-dose fluconazole treatment for oral or oesophageal infection. Many of these fluconazole-resistant *C. albicans* strains appear to be susceptible to other azoles. Resistant strains of *C. neoformans* have been recovered from patients with AIDS with relapsing cryptococcosis following long-term maintenance treatment with fluconazole, but this is an uncommon problem at present.

Three mechanisms of azole drug resistance have so far been recognized. The first is reduced intracellular drug accumulation. This results either from reduced drug uptake or from increased drug excretion. Recent work suggests that accelerated efflux of fluconazole, due to the action of multidrug resistance gene products, is the main reason for reduced drug access. The second resistance mechanism is structural alteration of the 14α-demethylase enzyme that results in decreased binding to azole antifungals. The third mechanism is overproduction of this target enzyme, due to gene amplification. The existence of multiple resistance mechanisms to agents with a common mode of action may explain why many fluconazole-resistant strains of *C. albicans* remain susceptible to other azoles.

3.3.4 Pharmacokinetics

Oral administration of fluconazole leads to rapid and almost complete absorption of the drug. Identical serum concentrations are attained after oral and parenteral administration indicating that first-pass metabolism of the drug does not occur. Blood concentrations increase in proportion to dosage over a wide range of dose levels. Two hours after a single 50-mg oral dose, serum concentrations in the region of 1.0 mg/l can be anticipated, but after repeated dosing this increases to about 2.0–3.0 mg/l. Administration of the drug with food does not affect absorption.

Oral or parenteral administration of fluconazole results in

rapid and widespread distribution of the drug. Unlike other azole antifungals, the protein binding of fluconazole is low (about 12%) resulting in high levels of circulating unbound drug. Levels of the drug in most tissues and fluids usually exceed 50% of the simultaneous blood concentration. The main means of elimination is renal excretion of the unchanged drug. About 80% of an administered dose appears in the urine in unchanged form and concentrations of > 100 mg/l have been attained in patients with normal renal function. The drug is cleared through glomerular filtration, but significant tubular reabsorption occurs. Fluconazole has a serum half-life of 20–30 h, but this is prolonged in renal failure, necessitating adjustment of the dosage regimen in patients with glomerular filtration rates below 50 ml/min.

Fluconazole is removed during haemodialysis and, to a lesser extent, during peritoneal dialysis. A 3-h haemodialysis session will reduce the blood concentration by about 50%.

3.3.5   **Metabolism**
Unlike other azole antifungals, fluconazole is not extensively metabolized in humans. More than 90% of a given dose is eliminated in the urine: about 80% as unchanged drug and 10% as metabolites. There is no indication of significant induction or inhibition of fluconazole metabolism following repeated dosing.

3.3.6   **Pharmaceutics**
Fluconazole is available in oral and parenteral forms: as capsules, oral suspension and an intravenous infusion. The drug is supplied for parenteral administration at a concentration of 2.0 mg/ml in 0.9% sodium chloride solution. Dosing recommendations are identical for all dosage forms.

3.3.7   **Therapeutic use**
Fluconazole can be used to treat mucosal and cutaneous forms of candidosis. It is also effective in various forms of dermatophytosis and pityriasis versicolor.

It is a promising drug for treatment of deep forms of candidosis in patients without neutropenia, but should not be used as first-line treatment in neutropenic patients unless there are particular reasons for favouring it against established management. Fluconazole has proved to be a useful prophylactic treatment against candidosis in neutropenic patients. However, it is ineffective in aspergillosis and mucormycosis.

Fluconazole is a useful drug in acute cryptococcal meningitis, but should not be used as first-line treatment in patients with AIDS unless there are particular reasons for withholding amphotericin B. However, it is more effective and better tolerated than amphotericin B as maintenance treatment to prevent relapse of cryptococcosis in patients with AIDS.

Fluconazole is now the drug of choice for patients with coccidioidal meningitis. However, it must be continued for life to prevent relapse.

3.3.8   ## Mode of administration

As absorption following oral administration is good, this is the preferred method of administration. If the patient cannot take the drug by mouth, the intravenous solution can be used. This should be infused at a rate of 5–10 ml/min.

Vaginal candidosis can be treated with a single 150-mg oral dose of fluconazole. Oropharyngeal candidosis should be treated with 50–200 mg/day for 1–2 weeks. Oesophageal and mucocutaneous forms of candidosis and lower urinary tract candidosis require 100–200 mg/day for 2–4 weeks.

The recommended dose for patients with cryptococcosis or deep forms of candidosis is 400 mg/day. However, some clinicians have used higher dosages in life-threatening infections. The duration of treatment will differ from patient to patient, depending upon the nature and extent of the infection and the underlying illness. At least 6–8 weeks is usually required for successful treatment of cryptococcosis in patients without AIDS. The recommended dose for children is 1–2 mg/kg for superficial forms of candidosis and 5 mg/kg for cryptococcosis or deep forms of candidosis.

Long-term maintenance treatment with fluconazole to prevent relapse in patients with AIDS with cryptococcosis should be administered at a dosage of 200 mg/day. To prevent candidosis in neutropenic patients, the dose should be 100–400 mg/day. Patients at high risk of developing a deep-seated infection should receive 400 mg/day and this should be commenced several days before the anticipated onset of neutropenia and continued for 1 week after the neutrophil count recovers to $1 \times 10^9/l$.

Patients with renal impairment should be given the normal dose for the first 48 h of treatment. Thereafter, in persons with a creatinine clearance of 21–40 ml/min, the dosage interval should be doubled to 48 h or the dose halved. Persons with a clearance of 10–20 ml/min require a 72-h interval between doses.

Patients receiving regular haemodialysis require the usual dose after each dialysis session.

3.3.9 Adverse reactions

Fluconazole is well tolerated. The most common side-effects are gastrointestinal in origin, such as nausea and abdominal discomfort, but these seldom necessitate discontinuation of treatment in patients receiving up to 400 mg/day. Transient asymptomatic elevations of serum transaminase levels are quite common in patients with AIDS treated with the drug, and treatment should be discontinued in patients who have symptomatic hepatitis or test findings indicative of progressive or persistent hepatic dysfunction.

Fatal exfoliative skin rashes (Stevens–Johnson syndrome) have been reported in patients with AIDS or cancer, but the causal relationship with fluconazole is unclear because of the concomitant administration of other drugs. It is advisable to discontinue fluconazole in a patient with a superficial fungal infection who develops a skin rash. Patients with deep-seated fungal infection who develop rashes should be monitored and the drug discontinued if bullous lesions or erythema multiforme develop.

Unlike ketoconazole, fluconazole, when given in recommended doses, does not inhibit human adrenal or testicular steroid metabolism.

3.3.10 Drug interactions

Most drug interactions with azole antifungals occur by means of one of two basic mechanisms: impairment of the absorption of the azole compound leading to reduced blood concentrations; or interference with hepatic microsomal enzymes which alters the metabolism and blood concentrations of the azole, the interacting drug, or both.

Unlike itraconazole and ketoconazole, absorption of fluconazole is not reduced if it is given together with drugs that reduce gastric acid secretion. Concomitant administration of fluconazole and rifampicin has resulted in a modest reduction in blood levels of the antifungal agent. The effect is less marked than with itraconazole or ketoconazole and is due to induction of P-450 cytochrome oxidases by rifampicin with resulting enhanced hepatic metabolism of the azole drug.

Like rifampicin, phenytoin undergoes cytochrome P-450-mediated hepatic metabolism and its concomitant administration with fluconazole may reduce its clearance. If these drugs are given together, serum concentrations of phenytoin should be monitored and the phenytoin dose adjusted to maintain therapeutic levels.

Fluconazole has been shown to prolong the serum half-life, thus augmenting the hypoglycaemic effects of drugs, such as chlorpropamide, glibenclamide, glipizide and tolbutamide. Fluconazole can also increase the serum concentration of warfarin, augmenting its anticoagulant effects. Careful monitoring of prothrombin time in patients receiving concomitant treatment with fluconazole and anticoagulants is recommended.

Fluconazole may prolong the half-life of cyclosporin in transplant recipients, leading to increased blood levels of that drug. Serum concentrations of cyclosporin should be monitored if these drugs are given together.

3.4 Flucytosine

Flucytosine (5-fluorocytosine) is a synthetic fluorinated pyrimidine.

3.4.1 Mechanism of action

Flucytosine is transported into susceptible fungal cells by the action of cytosine permease and there converted by cytosine deaminase to 5-fluorouracil which is incorporated into RNA in place of uracil, with resulting abnormalities of protein synthesis. In addition, it blocks thymidylate synthetase causing inhibition of DNA synthesis.

3.4.2 Spectrum of action

Flucytosine has a limited spectrum of action including *Candida* species, *Cryptococcus neoformans*, *Cladosporium carrionii* (now reclassified as *Cladophialophora carrionii*), *Fonsecaea* species and *Phialophora verrucosa*.

3.4.3 Acquired resistance

Induction of resistance during treatment is a common problem. Moreover, about 10% of C. *albicans* strains, 20% of C. *tropicalis* strains and 2% of C. *neoformans* strains are resistant from the outset. The most common cause of resistance appears to be loss of the enzyme uridine monophosphate pyrophosphorylase.

3.4.4 Pharmacokinetics

Oral administration of flucytosine leads to rapid and almost complete absorption of the drug. Identical serum concentrations are obtained after oral and parenteral administration. In adults with normal renal function an oral dose of 25 mg/kg given at 6-h intervals will produce peak serum concentrations at 1–2 h of 70–80 mg/l and trough concentrations of 30–40 mg/l. Absorption is slower in persons with impaired renal function but peak serum concentrations are higher. There is slight accumulation of the drug during the first 4 days of treatment, but thereafter peak serum concentrations remain almost constant. Peak levels are reached in a shorter period of 1–2 h in persons who have received several previous doses of the drug. The protein binding of flucytosine is low (about 12%) resulting in high levels of circulating unbound drug.

Flucytosine is widely distributed, with levels in most tissues and fluids usually exceeding 50% of the simultaneous blood concentration. The main means of elimination is renal excretion of the unchanged drug. About 90% of an administered dose appears in the urine and concentrations of 1000 mg/l are not unusual in persons with normal renal function. The serum half-life is between 3 and 6 h, but is much longer in renal failure, necessitating modification of the dosage regimen.

3.4.5 Metabolism

Less than 1% of an administered dose of flucytosine is metabolized in humans. The drug is deaminated to 5-fluorouracil or dihydrofluorouracil and this could account for the myelotoxic effects associated with high serum concentrations. The remainder of the compound is excreted unchanged in the urine.

3.4.6   Pharmaceutics

Flucytosine is available as oral tablets and as an infusion for parenteral administration. The latter is supplied in 250-ml amounts containing 10 mg/ml in aqueous saline solution.

3.4.7   Therapeutic use

Flucytosine is seldom used as a single drug, other than in patients with certain forms of chromoblastomycosis. Its principal use is in combination with amphotericin B in the treatment of cryptococcosis and deep forms of candidosis. Flucytosine may be useful in combination with fluconazole or itraconazole in the treatment of acute cryptococcal meningitis in patients with AIDS.

3.4.8   Mode of administration

As absorption following oral administration is good this is the preferred method of administration. If the patient cannot take the drug by mouth, the intravenous solution should be used. This can be administered through a venous catheter or as an intraperitoneal infusion. The drug should be infused over a 20–40-min period provided this is balanced with the fluid requirements of the patient. Twice weekly blood counts (total white cells and platelets) should be performed.

In adults with normal renal function the usual starting dose of flucytosine is 50–150 mg/kg given as four divided doses at 6-h intervals. If renal function is impaired, an initial dose of 25 mg/kg should be given, but the subsequent dose and interval should be adjusted so as to produce peak serum concentrations of 70–80 mg/l and trough concentrations of 30–40 mg/l. The drug accumulates in renal failure necessitating modification of the dose regimen (Table 3.3). The half-life of flucytosine is prolonged in small infants and the drug should be administered at 12-or 24-h intervals.

3.4.9   Adverse reactions

Nausea, vomiting and diarrhoea are the most common side-effects. Thrombocytopenia and leucopenia can occur if excessive blood concentrations are maintained (more than 100 mg/l). The effect is usually reversible if treatment is discontinued. Bone marrow suppression is a common problem in patients with AIDS and usage of flucytosine should be minimized or avoided in these individuals.

Table 3.3 Regimens for administration of flucytosine in renal impairment.

Creatinine clearance (ml/min)	Individual dosage (mg/kg)	Dosage interval (h)
>40	25–37.5	6
40–20	25–37.5	12
20–10	25–37.5	24
<10	25–37.5	>24*

Renal function is considered to be normal when creatinine clearance is greater than 40–50 ml/min or concentration of creatinine in serum is less than 180 μmol/l; concentration of creatinine in serum is not reliable unless renal function is stable.
* Dosage interval must be based on serum drug concentration measurement at frequent intervals.

Elevated transaminase levels develop in some patients, but usually return to normal after the drug is discontinued. Liver necrosis leading or contributing to death has been reported in occasional patients.

3.4.10 Drug interactions

Amphotericin B and flucytosine have an additive or synergistic effect when used in combination against *Candida* species and *C. neoformans*. However, the nephrotoxic effects of amphotericin B result in elevated blood levels of flucytosine and concentrations of the latter drug should be monitored when these compounds are administered together.

There have been a number of reports of successful treatment of candidosis and cryptococcosis with combinations of flucytosine and fluconazole or itraconazole. The results of comparative clinical trials are awaited.

3.5 Griseofulvin

Griseofulvin is an antifungal antibiotic derived from a number of *Penicillium* species. It was the first oral drug for treatment of dermatophytosis.

3.5.1 Mechanism of action

Griseofulvin is a fungistatic drug which binds to microtubular proteins and inhibits fungal cell mitosis. It also acts as an inhibitor of nucleic acid synthesis.

3.5.2 Spectrum of action

Griseofulvin has a limited spectrum of action which is almost restricted to the dermatophytes (*Epidermophyton floccosum*, *Microsporum* species and *Trichophyton* species). Its clinical use is limited to these infections. It is ineffective in cutaneous candidosis and pityriasis versicolor.

3.5.3 Acquired resistance

Treatment failure attributable to the development of griseofulvin resistance is an uncommon problem in patients with dermatophytoses.

3.5.4 Pharmacokinetics

Absorption of griseofulvin from the gastrointestinal tract is dependent on drug formulation. Administration of the drug with a high fat meal will increase the rate and extent of absorption, but individual patients tend to achieve consistently high or low serum concentrations. Four hours after a single 1000-mg dose, blood levels in the region of 0–3.75 mg/l can be anticipated.

Griseofulvin appears in the stratum corneum within 4–8 h of oral administration, as a result of drug secretion in perspiration. However, levels begin to fall soon after the drug is discontinued and within 48–72 h it can no longer be detected. The mechanisms by which griseofulvin is delivered to the hair and nails are not well understood: deposition in newly formed cells is thought to be the major factor.

3.5.5 Metabolism

Griseofulvin is metabolized by the liver to 6-desmethyl griseofulvin which is excreted in the urine. The drug has an elimination half-life from 9 to 21 h. Less than 1% of a given dose appears in the urine in unchanged form.

3.5.6 Pharmaceutics

Griseofulvin is available as oral tablets and oral suspension.

3.5.7 Therapeutic use

Griseofulvin is indicated in moderate to severe dermatophytoses of the skin, scalp hair, or nails where topical treatment is considered inappropriate or has failed.

3.5.8   **Mode of administration**
It is important to adjust the dose to the weight of the patient. The adult dose can range from 500 to 1000 mg either as a single or divided doses; not less than 10 mg/kg should be given. The dose for children under 25 kg is 10 mg/kg and 250–500 mg for children over 25 kg. It should be taken after meals.

The duration of treatment will differ from patient to patient and depend upon the nature and extent of the infection. For hair or skin at least 4 weeks of treatment is required. Long courses (usually 6–12 months) and high doses may be needed for nail infections. Long-term relapse rates are high; between 40 and 70% for toenails, but somewhat lower for fingernails.

3.5.9   **Adverse reactions**
In most cases, prolonged courses and high doses are well tolerated. Patients have complained of headaches, nausea, vomiting and abdominal discomfort. Urticarial reactions and erythematous rashes occur in occasional patients.

The drug is contraindicated in patients with liver disease as hepatic function may deteriorate and the risk of other side-effects is increased.

3.5.10   **Drug interactions**
Griseofulvin has been shown to stimulate the metabolism of warfarin, thus reducing its anticoagulant effect. Absorption is reduced in patients receiving concomitant treatment with phenobarbitone, but the effect can be reduced by administration of griseofulvin with food. Failure of contraception has been reported in patients taking griseofulvin and oral contraceptive steroids.

3.6   **Itraconazole**
Itraconazole is a synthetic dioxolane triazole compound.

3.6.1   **Mechanism of action**
Like other azoles, it interferes with the cytochrome P-450-dependent enzyme, 14α-demethylase. This leads to 14-methylsterol accumulation and ergosterol depletion in

fungal cells and this results in alterations in a number of membrane-associated cell functions.

3.6.2 Spectrum of action

Itraconazole has a broad spectrum of action including *Aspergillus* species, *Blastomyces dermatitidis*, *Candida* species, *Coccidioides immitis*, *Cryptococcus neoformans*, *Histoplasma capsulatum*, *Paracoccidioides brasiliensis*, *Scedosporium apiospermum* and *Sporothrix schenckii*. It is active in dermatophytosis and pityriasis versicolor, but appears to be ineffective in mucormycosis.

3.6.3 Acquired resistance

This is rare, but ketoconazole-resistant *C. albicans* strains from patients with chronic mucocutaneous candidosis have been cross-resistant to itraconazole, as have some fluconazole-resistant *C. albicans* strains from patients with AIDS with chronic relapsing oropharyngeal candidosis.

3.6.4 Pharmacokinetics

Absorption of itraconazole from the gastrointestinal tract is incomplete (about 55%), but is improved if the drug is given with food. Oral administration of a single 100-mg capsule will produce peak serum concentrations of between 0.1 and 0.2 mg/l about 2–4 h later. Higher concentrations are obtained after repeated dosing, but there is marked variation between individuals. As with ketoconazole, there is a disproportionate increase in blood levels with increasing dosage. Serum concentrations are markedly reduced when gastric acid production is impaired.

Much higher blood concentrations (up to 1.0–1.5 mg/l) have been attained in patients with AIDS and neutropenic individuals following administration of a 5 mg/kg dose of the oral solution formulation of itraconazole for 1–2 weeks. This formulation is better absorbed if given without food.

Like most other azole antifungals, the protein binding of itraconazole is high, exceeding 99% in human serum. As a result, concentrations of the drug in body fluids such as CSF are minimal. In contrast, drug concentrations in tissues, such as lung, liver and bone, are two to three times higher than in serum. High concentrations of itraconazole are also found in the stratum corneum as a result of drug secretion in

sebum. Itraconazole has been found to persist in the skin for 2–4 weeks after the end of a 4-week course of treatment. It persists in toenails for up to 6 months after the end of a 3-month course of treatment, but levels in the fingernails decline about 3 months after the end of treatment.

Less than 0.03% of an administered dose of itraconazole is excreted unchanged in the urine, but up to 18% is eliminated in faeces as unchanged drug.

3.6.5 Metabolism

Itraconazole is degraded by the liver into a large number of metabolites, most of which are inactive and these are excreted with the bile and urine. However, the major metabolite, hydroxyitraconazole, is bioactive. The serum half-life is about 20–30 h, increasing to 40 h after prolonged dosing.

3.6.6 Pharmaceutics

Itraconazole is available as oral capsules and oral solution.

3.6.7 Therapeutic use

Itraconazole can be used to treat various superficial fungal infections, including the dermatophytoses, pityriasis versicolor, and mucosal and cutaneous forms of candidosis. It is also effective in patients with subcutaneous infections, such as chromoblastomycosis, sporotrichosis and certain forms of phaeohyphomycosis. It has become the drug of choice for non-life-threatening forms of blastomycosis and histoplasmosis, and is a useful alternative to amphotericin B for invasive aspergillosis. Maintenance treatment with itraconazole has helped to prevent relapse in patients with AIDS with histoplasmosis or cryptococcosis, and prophylactic treatment with this drug has helped to prevent aspergillosis and candidosis in neutropenic patients. However, it has not been adequately evaluated as an oral treatment for deep-seated forms of candidosis.

3.6.8 Mode of administration

Vaginal candidosis can be treated with two 200-mg oral doses of itraconazole taken 6–8 h apart. In non-compromised individuals, oropharyngeal candidosis can be treated with 100 mg/day for 2 weeks, but neutropenic patients and those with AIDS often require 200–400 mg/day

because of impaired oral absorption. Administering the oral solution formulation (200–400 mg/day for 1–2 weeks) often results in improved absorption.

The recommended dosage for patients with cutaneous dermatophytoses is 100 mg/day, but the duration of treatment depends on the site of infection. Tinea corporis or tinea cruris should be treated for 2 weeks, but tinea pedis and tinea manuum require treatment for 4 weeks. Pulsed treatment (in which a week of treatment is alternated with 3 weeks without treatment) has given good results in nail infections. Two pulses of itraconazole (400 mg/day) are recommended for fingernail infections, but toenails require three or more pulses of treatment. Itraconazole is also available for continuous treatment of nail infection and a dosage of 200 mg/day for 3 months is recommended.

The recommended dosage for patients with pityriasis versicolor is 200 mg/day for 1 week.

Itraconazole, at dosages from 200 to 400 mg/day, is usually effective in patients with subcutaneous or deep fungal infection. Some clinicians have used loading doses of 600 mg/day at the start of treatment in patients with life-threatening infections. Impaired absorption in neutropenic patients and those with AIDS will lead to low blood levels and higher dosages, or substitution of the oral solution formulation, may be required to ensure adequate serum concentrations. Absorption of itraconazole is reduced if it is given together with compounds that reduce gastric acid secretion: these drugs should be administered at least 2 h after the intake of itraconazole. Dosages above 200 mg/day should be given as two divided doses.

Long-term maintenance treatment with itraconazole to prevent relapse in patients with AIDS with histoplasmosis or cryptococcosis should be administered at a dosage of 200 mg/day. To prevent fungal infection in neutropenic patients, the dose should be 400 mg/day and this should be commenced about 5–7 days before the anticipated onset of neutropenia.

3.6.9 Adverse reactions

Itraconazole is well tolerated. The most frequently reported side-effects are gastrointestinal in origin, such as nausea, abdominal discomfort and constipation. Less common side-effects include headache, dizziness, pruritus and allergic

rashes. Isolated cases of Stevens–Johnson syndrome have been reported.

Transient asymptomatic elevations of serum transaminase levels have been reported and the drug is best avoided in patients with liver disease and those who have experienced hepatotoxic reactions with other drugs, unless the expected benefit outweighs the risk. In such cases, monitoring of liver function is essential.

Unlike ketoconazole, itraconazole, when given in recommended doses, has no effect on human adrenal or testicular steroid metabolism.

3.6.10 Drug interactions

Absorption of itraconazole is reduced if it is given together with drugs that reduce gastric acid secretion, such as antacids, H2-antagonists, omeprazole and lansoprazole. Concomitant administration with enzyme-inducing drugs, such as phenytoin and rifampicin, results in a marked reduction in blood levels of itraconazole.

Itraconazole has been shown to inhibit the metabolism, thus prolonging the half-life of terfenadine, astemizole and cisapride, predisposing patients to serious cardiac arrhythmias. Itraconazole should not be administered concomitantly with these drugs.

Itraconazole can also prolong the half-life of midazolam and triazolam, thus augmenting their serum concentrations. It should not be administered concomitantly with these drugs.

Itraconazole has been shown to increase the serum concentrations of digoxin and cyclosporin and levels of these drugs should be monitored if they are given together with itraconazole. Itraconazole can also increase the serum concentration of warfarin, enhancing its anticoagulant effect. Careful monitoring of prothrombin time in patients receiving both drugs is recommended.

Co-administration of itraconazole and vincristine may potentiate the toxic effects of the latter drug and, should this occur, itraconazole treatment may need to be discontinued.

3.7 Ketoconazole

Ketoconazole is a synthetic dioxolane imidazole compound.

3.7.1   **Mechanism of action**
Like other azoles, it interferes with the biosynthesis of ergosterol, leading to alterations in a number of membrane-associated cell functions.

3.7.2   **Spectrum of action**
It has a broad spectrum of action including *Blastomyces dermatitidis*, *Candida* species, *Coccidioides immitis*, *Histoplasma capsulatum* and *Paracoccidioides brasiliensis*. It is active in dermatophytosis and pityriasis versicolor, but ineffective in aspergillosis and mucormycosis.

3.7.3   **Acquired resistance**
This is rare, but resistant *C. albicans* strains have been recovered from patients treated for chronic mucocutaneous candidosis and patients with AIDS with chronic relapsing oropharyngeal candidosis. Some fluconazole-resistant *C. albicans* strains from patients with AIDS are cross-resistant to ketoconazole.

3.7.4   **Pharmacokinetics**
Ketoconazole is not absorbed after topical application, but is well absorbed after oral administration, peak serum concentrations being reached 2–4 h later. Food delays absorption but does not significantly reduce the peak concentration. Two hours after a 400-mg dose serum concentrations in the region of 5–6 mg/l can be anticipated, but there is much variation among individuals. Much higher concentrations can be obtained with doses of 600–1000 mg. Penetration into CSF is poor and unreliable, although effective concentrations have been recorded with high doses (1200 mg) in some cases of meningitis. Less than 1% of an oral dose is excreted unchanged in the urine.

3.7.5   **Metabolism**
The drug is metabolized in the liver and the metabolites are excreted in the bile. None of the metabolites are active. The half-life appears to be dose-dependent. There is an initial half-life of 1–4 h and an elimination half-life ranging from 6 to 10 h.

3.7.6   **Pharmaceutics**
It is available in a number of oral and topical forms.

3.7.7 **Therapeutic use**

Until the introduction of fluconazole and itraconazole, ketoconazole was regarded as the drug of choice for chronic mucocutaneous candidosis and an effective alternative treatment for certain forms of histoplasmosis, blastomycosis and paracoccidioidomycosis. However, prolonged administration of high dosage was often required and later relapse was a common problem. Ketoconazole has not been adequately evaluated in deep-seated candidosis or cryptococcosis and it is ineffective in aspergillosis and mucormycosis. It should not be used for the oral treatment of dermatophytosis or cutaneous or vaginal candidosis, because of its possible effects on the liver and on steroid metabolism. However, it is a useful topical drug for dermatophytosis, cutaneous candidosis, pityriasis versicolor and seborrhoeic dermatitis.

3.7.8 **Mode of administration**

Topical ketoconazole cream should be applied morning and evening and treatment should be continued for 48 h after all symptoms and signs have cleared. Pityriasis versicolor and sebhorrhoeic dermatitis can be treated with ketoconazole shampoo.

The usual adult oral dose is 200–400 mg/day depending on the infection being treated. In children a dose of 3 mg/kg can be used. The duration of treatment will depend upon the nature of the infection.

Absorption of ketoconazole is reduced if it is given together with drugs that reduce gastric acid secretion. If patients are receiving antacids, anticholinergics or H2-antagonists, these should be given at least 2 h after ketoconazole administration.

3.7.9 **Adverse reactions**

Anorexia, nausea and vomiting are the most common side-effects. These dose-related effects occur in up to 50% of patients receiving oral doses of > 800 mg, but taking the drug with food or at bedtime may improve tolerance.

Mild hepatotoxic effects are common with oral ketoconazole, but serious liver damage is rare. Transient transaminase elevations occur in about 5–10% of patients on oral ketoconazole. Treatment must be discontinued if these persist, if the abnormalities increase, or if symptoms associated with hepatic dysfunction appear. The serious hepatotoxic side-effects of ketoconazole are idiosyncratic and rare, occurring in between 1:10 000 and 1:15 000 patients treated for longer than 2 weeks. Most cases have been reported in patients treated for onychomycosis or chronic recalcitrant dermatophytosis. In most cases, hepatic damage is reversible when the drug is discontinued. Liver function tests should be performed before starting treatment and at monthly intervals thereafter, particularly in patients on prolonged treatment or in those receiving other hepatotoxic drugs.

High doses of ketoconazole (over 800 mg/day) inhibit human adrenal and testicular steroid synthesis, with clinical consequences such as alopecia, gynaecomastia and impotence. High-dose ketoconazole should be avoided in conditions associated with hypoadrenalism: these include AIDS, histoplasmosis, paracoccidioidomycosis and tuberculosis.

3.7.10 Drug interactions

As with itraconazole, serum concentrations of ketoconazole are lower in patients taking drugs that reduce gastric acid secretion, such as antacids, anticholinergics and H2-antagonists. Concurrent administration of ketoconazole with rifampicin may reduce the effectiveness of both drugs.

Oral ketoconazole has been shown to prolong the half-life of terfenadine, astemizole and cisapride, predisposing patients to serious cardiac arrhythmias. It should not be administered concomitantly with these drugs. Ketoconazole can also prolong the half-life of midazolam and triazolam, thus augmenting their serum concentrations. It has been shown to increase the blood levels of cyclosporin and levels of this drug should be monitored if it is given together with this antifungal agent. Ketoconazole can also increase the serum concentration of warfarin, enhancing its anticoagulant effect. Careful monitoring of prothrombin time in patients receiving both drugs is recommended.

3.8 Miconazole

Miconazole is a synthetic phenethyl imidazole compound.

3.8.1 Mechanism of action

Like other azoles, it interferes with the biosynthesis of

ergosterol, leading to alterations in a number of membrane-associated cell functions. At high concentrations, miconazole interacts with membrane lipids causing direct membrane damage which results in leakage of cell constituents.

3.8.2 Spectrum of action

Miconazole has a limited spectrum of action including *Candida* species, *Coccidioides immitis*, *Histoplasma capsulatum*, *Paracoccidioides brasiliensis* and *Scedosporium apiospermum*. It is also active in dermatophytosis.

3.8.3 Acquired resistance

This is rare but *C. albicans* strains resistant to ketoconazole have been cross-resistant to miconazole.

3.8.4 Pharmacokinetics

Miconazole is poorly absorbed following oral administration. Parenteral administration of a single 1000-mg dose will produce peak serum concentrations up to 7.5 mg/l. There is rapid decline, with an initial serum half-life of 20–30 min and an elimination half-life of about 20 h.

Miconazole is highly protein-bound in serum. Concentrations in CSF are poor, but there is good penetration into peritoneal and joint fluid, and aqueous and vitreous humour. Less than 1% of a parenteral dose is excreted unchanged in the urine, but 40% of an oral dose is eliminated in faeces as unchanged drug.

3.8.5 Metabolism

Miconazole is metabolized by the liver and the metabolites are excreted in the bile and urine. None of the metabolites is active.

3.8.6 Pharmaceutics

Miconazole base is available in oral and parenteral forms. Miconazole nitrate is supplied in several forms for topical application.

The drug is supplied for parenteral administration in 20-ml amounts of cremophor containing 10 mg/ml. It must be diluted with sodium chloride solution or 5% dextrose solution.

3.8.7 **Therapeutic use**

Topical miconazole can be used to treat the dermatophytoses, and cutaneous and mucosal candidosis. Parenteral miconazole has been used to treat coccidioidomycosis and paracoccidioidomycosis. However, failure and relapse have been a frequent problem. Its role in cryptococcosis and deep forms of candidosis remains unclear and it cannot now be recommended for these infections. It is ineffective in aspergillosis and mucormycosis, but is more active than amphotericin B in *Scedosporium apiospermum* (*Pseudallescheria boydii*) infection.

3.8.8 **Mode of administration**

Vaginal candidosis can be treated with a 5-g dose of miconazole each night for 2 weeks, or 10 g can be administered for 1 week. For those with cutaneous dematophytosis, topical miconazole should be applied morning and evening until 2 weeks after the lesions have cleared. Cream containing miconazole nitrate and a steroid is useful in reducing inflammation.

The optimum dosage regimens for specific deep fungal infections or sites of infection have not been established. The usual adult dose is 600 mg given at 8-h intervals over a period of not less than 30 min, but doses as high as 1200 mg per infusion have been used. Rapid infusion of miconazole must be avoided. The duration of treatment will depend upon the infection and the underlying illness of the patient.

3.8.9 **Adverse reactions**

Topical miconazole can cause local irritation. Oral forms of the drug have caused mild gastrointestinal upsets. Parenteral miconazole is associated with a number of serious adverse reactions associated with the drug itself or the vehicle. Miconazole itself causes nausea, vomiting and hyponatraemia. The vehicle causes histamine release and induces intense pruritus, necessitating discontinuation of the drug in some patients. Infusion of the drug is often associated with local phlebitis at peripheral injection sites.

Rapid injection of miconazole can produce transient tachycardia or cardiac arrhythmia. These effects, if not transient, respond to lignocaine.

3.8.10   **Drug interactions**
Like other azoles, miconazole can affect the clearance of
drugs that undergo cytochrome P-450-dependent hepatic
metabolism. It should not be administered concomitantly
with terfenadine, astemizole or cisapride because of the risk
of ventricular arrhythmias. Miconazole can also increase the
serum concentration of warfarin, augmenting its anticoagulant effect.

3.9   **Terbinafine**
Terbinafine is a synthetic allylamine compound.

3.9.1   **Mechanism of action**
Terbinafine inhibits the action of squalene epoxidase, a
crucial enzyme in the formation of ergosterol, the principal
sterol in the membrane of susceptible fungal cells. The
consequent accumulation of squalene leads to membrane
disruption and cell death.

3.9.2   **Spectrum of action**
Terbinafine is effective against the dermatophytes
(*Epidermophyton floccosum*, *Microsporum* species and
Trichophyton species) and *Malassezia furfur*. It is fungistatic for *Candida albicans* but fungicidal for some other
Candida species including *C. parapsilosis*. It has also been
shown to be active against *Aspergillus* species, and its
clinical effectiveness against these and other systemic and
subcutaneous pathogens is now under investigation.

3.9.3   **Acquired resistance**
This has not been reported.

3.9.4   **Pharmacokinetics**
About 5% of a given dose of terbinafine is absorbed following topical application. The drug is well absorbed
(> 70%) after oral administration, peak serum concentrations in the region of 0.8–1.5 mg/l being attained 2 h after a
single 250-mg dose. Levels increase in proportion to dosage
up to at least 750 mg. Administration of the drug with food
does not affect absorption.
    Terbinafine is a lipophilic drug which appears to con-
centrate in the dermis, epidermis and adipose tissue. It
appears in the stratum corneum within a few hours of oral

administration being commenced, as a result of diffusion through the dermis and epidermis and secretion in sebum. Diffusion from the nail bed is the major factor in its rapid penetration of nails. Terbinafine has been found to persist in nail for long periods after cessation of treatment.

3.9.5 Metabolism

Terbinafine is metabolized by the liver and the inactive metabolites are excreted in the urine. The drug has an elimination half-life of 17 h, but this is prolonged in patients with hepatic or renal impairment.

3.9.6 Pharmaceutics

Terbinafine (as hydrochloride) is available in oral and topical forms.

3.9.7 Therapeutic use

Topical terbinafine is effective against cutaneous dermatophytoses and candidosis, as well as pityriasis versicolor. Oral terbinafine can be used to treat dermatophytoses of the skin and nails where topical treatment is considered inappropriate or has failed. However, oral treatment is ineffective against pityriasis versicolor.

3.9.8 Mode of administration

Topical terbinafine should be applied morning and/or evening for 2–4 weeks depending on the site of infection. Tinea pedis should be treated for 2 weeks, and tinea corporis and cruris for 2–4 weeks. Cutaneous candidosis and pityriasis versicolor should be treated for 2 weeks.

The usual adult dose of oral terbinafine is 250 mg/day, but this should be halved in patients with impaired hepatic or renal function (creatinine clearance less than 50 ml/min or serum creatinine concentration > 300 μmol/ml). The duration of treatment will depend upon the site and extent of infection (see Chapter 4). Tinea pedis should be treated for 2–6 weeks, and tinea corporis and cruris for 2–4 weeks. Most nail infections require at least 6 weeks of oral terbinafine treatment. Fingernail infection can often be cured with treatment periods of less than 3 months, but some patients with toenail infection require treatment for 6 months or longer.

3.9.9 **Adverse reactions**

Terbinafine is well tolerated. The most common side-effects are gastrointestinal in origin, such as nausea and mild abdominal pain. Allergic skin reactions have also been reported and isolated cases of Stevens–Johnson syndrome have occurred. If a progressive skin rash develops which is considered to be attributable to terbinafine, the drug should be discontinued. Taste loss and taste disturbance have been reported, but these usually resolve slowly once the drug is stopped.

Occasional cases of serious hepatic dysfunction, including cholestasis and hepatitis have been reported. Should this occur, treatment with terbinafine should be discontinued.

3.9.10 **Drug interactions**

Unlike the azole antifungals, terbinafine does not affect the clearance of drugs, such as cyclosporin and tolbutamide, that undergo cytochrome P-450-dependent hepatic metabolism. However, blood concentrations of terbinafine are reduced following its concomitant administration with drugs, such as rifampicin, which induce hepatic metabolism. Blood levels are increased if terbinafine is given together with drugs, such as cimetidine, that inhibit cytochrome P-450-mediated hepatic metabolism.

3.10 **Other compounds for topical administration**

In addition to the antifungal compounds described so far, a number of other drugs are available for topical use.

3.10.1 **Amorolfine**

Morpholine compound which inhibits fungal ergosterol biosynthesis. It can be used to treat localized distal nail disease due to dermatophytosis, candidosis, or mould infection. Amorolfine should be applied at 1-week intervals for at least 6 months for fingernail infection and 12 months for toenail infection.

3.10.2 **Bifonazole**

Imidazole compound used for the treatment of the dermatophytoses and pityriasis versicolor.

3.10.3 **Clotrimazole**

Imidazole compound used for the treatment of the dermatophytoses and oral, cutaneous and genital candidosis.

3.10.4 **Econazole nitrate**

Imidazole compound used for the treatment of the dermatophytoses and oral, cutaneous and genital candidosis. It has also been used to treat corneal infections.

3.10.5 **Isoconazole nitrate**

Imidazole compound used for the treatment of vaginal candidosis.

3.10.6 **Naftifine**

Allylamine compound used for the treatment of the dermatophytoses.

3.10.7 **Natamycin**

Polyene compound used for the treatment of oral and vaginal candidosis. It has also been used to treat corneal infections.

3.10.8 **Nystatin**

Polyene compound used for the treatment of oral, cutaneous and mucosal forms of candidosis. It has also been used to treat corneal infections.

3.10.9 **Sulconazole nitrate**

Imidazole compound used for the treatment of the dermatophytoses and cutaneous candidosis.

3.10.10 **Tioconazole**

Imidazole compound used for the treatment of the dermatophytoses (including nail infections) and cutaneous and vaginal candidosis.

3.11 **Empirical treatment of suspected fungal infection in the neutropenic patient**

Treatment of established candidosis or aspergillosis in the neutropenic patient is often unsuccessful. For this reason it is often better to begin antifungal treatment without waiting for formal proof that a neutropenic patient with persistent fever (greater than 72–96 h duration), resistant to broad-spectrum antibacterial agents, has a fungal infection. In this situation amphotericin B must be used. Should the conventional formulation be contraindicated, one of the lipid-based formulations should be used instead.

Empirical treatment should be initiated with the usual test dose (1 mg) of amphotericin B. If possible, the full therapeutic dosage level (1.0 mg/kg per day of the conventional formulation) should be reached within the first 24 h of treatment. There is no need for gradual escalation of dosage, nor is there evidence to support the clinical prejudice that a lower dose can be used in suspected candidosis.

The duration of treatment will differ from patient to patient. If the patient responds and a diagnosis of fungal infection is established, a full course of treatment should be given. More often, however, the patient responds and/or the neutrophil count recovers, but a firm diagnosis is not obtained. In this situation it is reasonable to discontinue amphotericin B when the neutrophil count exceeds 1×10^9/l, the fever resolves, other relevant symptoms and signs resolve, and relevant radiological abnormalities return to normal. Although there is no direct evidence to support the clinical prejudice that suspected aspergillosis requires a longer period of treatment than suspected candidosis, this common practice is justified.

Neutropenic patients who recover from a deep fungal infection, such as aspergillosis, may suffer from reactivation of the infection during subsequent periods of immunosuppression. One solution to this problem is to begin empirical treatment with amphotericin B (1 mg/kg per day) not less than 48 h before antileukaemic treatment is commenced. This drug should be continued until the neutrophil count has recovered.

3.12 Prophylactic treatment for prevention of fungal infection

There have been numerous attempts to develop regimens that will reduce intestinal and oral colonization with *Candida* species and help prevent oral candidosis. There have, however, been no convincing demonstrations that either nystatin or amphotericin B oral suspensions or tablets prevent the development of oral, oesophageal or deep forms of candidosis in immunocompromised patients. Their use alone is not recommended.

Oral ketoconazole does appear to reduce the incidence of oral candidosis and oesophagitis in neutropenic patients; whether it prevents deep candidosis is less clear. It offers no protection against aspergillosis or mucormycosis and its use can lead to the selection of less sensitive *C. glabrata* strains in the gastrointestinal tract. It is not well absorbed in bone marrow transplant (BMT) recipients. Moreover, it prolongs the half-life of cyclosporin and leads to increased serum concentrations of that drug. Its use as prophylaxis in organ transplant or BMT recipients is therefore not recommended.

Oral fluconazole (100–200 mg/day) has been shown to reduce the incidence of mucosal colonization and superficial infection with all *Candida* species apart from *C. glabrata* and *C. krusei*. However, it offers no protection against aspergillosis or mucormycosis. Those at high risk of developing a serious *Candida* infection should receive 400 mg/day. Fluconazole has much less effect on cyclosporin metabolism than other azoles and it can be recommended as an effective drug for prevention of candidosis in immunocompromised patients. However, it is prudent to measure cyclosporin levels if these drugs are given together.

Itraconazole does appear to help prevent the development of aspergillosis and candidosis in neutropenic patients. The introduction of an oral solution formulation has reduced the problem of erratic absorption of the drug from the gastrointestinal tract in BMT recipients and patients undergoing remission induction. Itraconazole, at a dosage of 400 mg/day, can be recommended as prophylaxis in units where patients are nursed without high efficiency particulate air (HEPA) filters, where there is a high incidence of aspergillosis, or where building works are being undertaken. It should be substituted for fluconazole prophylaxis in such institutions in patients who have been neutropenic for longer than 3 weeks.

3.13   Laboratory monitoring
3.13.1   Amphotericin B

The results of susceptibility tests with amphotericin B are less subject to test conditions than is the case with most other antifungal drugs. Most strains of most of the principal human pathogens are inhibited from growth at concentrations ranging from 0.05 to 1.0 mg/l. These concentrations are similar to blood levels attained during parenteral treatment, but it is unsafe to assume that all patients will respond to the drug. Other factors, such as the immunological status of the patient and the location of the infection, must be taken into account. There is usually no need to test isolates of *Aspergillus* species, *Candida* species or *C. neoformans* before starting treatment, because insensitive strains are rare. Isolates from patients with a serious infection that does not respond as expected to amphotericin B should be tested. Susceptibility tests with other moulds are sometimes helpful, but clinical correlations are not well established.

Routine monitoring of amphotericin B serum concentrations during treatment is not indicated. The question of the optimum serum concentration of the drug for a particular fungal infection has not been resolved. Although amphotericin B is nephrotoxic, high blood concentrations do not lead to greater impairment of renal function, nor does renal failure result in higher blood concentrations.

3.13.2 Fluconazole

As with other azoles, the results of susceptibility tests with fluconazole are highly dependent on the conditions, being markedly affected by the concentration of the fungal inoculum, the composition and pH of the medium, and the temperature and length of incubation. However, with the advent of standardized methods, these tests are becoming much more reliable in predicting clinical outcome in patients with candidosis and cryptococcosis.

Isolates from patients destined to receive fluconazole must be identified, as should isolates from cases of suspected treatment failure or relapse. Most *C. krusei* and *C. glabrata* isolates are resistant to fluconazole and the drug should not be used to treat infections with these organisms. Conversely, it is rare for *C. albicans* or *C. neoformans* to become resistant unless a patient has received one or more courses of azole treatment over a period of several months or longer. However, if treatment failure or relapse occur despite adequate serum concentrations of fluconazole, the minimum inhibitory concentration (MIC) of the drug for recent isolates from the patient should be compared with those of earlier isolates and susceptible and resistant reference organisms.

In general, serum concentrations of fluconazole are more predictable than those of other azole drugs and there is no need for their measurement. Excessive concentrations have not so far been associated with unwanted side-effects. Concentrations are unchanged in patients with AIDS and in BMT recipients, and the reduction in concentration following concomitant administration with rifampicin is smaller than that seen with other azole antifungals.

3.13.3 Flucytosine

The major disadvantage of this drug is the fact that a significant proportion of *C. albicans* and *C. neoformans* isolates are resistant with MICs in excess of 16 mg/l. For this reason, isolates from all patients destined to receive the drug on its own should be tested as should isolates recovered during treatment.

Serum concentrations of flucytosine should be measured in all patients; this is essential when there is renal impairment or when the drug is given in combination with amphotericin B, to ensure adequate therapeutic concentrations and avoid excessive concentrations that can cause toxic effects.

Levels should be determined twice weekly or more frequently if renal function is changing. Blood should be taken just before a dose of flucytosine is due, and 2 h after an oral dose or 30 min after an intravenous dose. In patients with renal impairment peak concentrations tend to occur later after oral dosing.

3.13.4 Itraconazole

As with fluconazole, the results of susceptibility tests are highly dependent on the conditions under which the tests are performed. However, with the advent of standardized methods, these tests are becoming much more reliable in predicting clinical outcome in patients with candidosis and cryptococcosis. Susceptibility tests with moulds are sometimes helpful, but clinical correlations are not well established.

Absorption of itraconazole after oral administration shows marked variation between individuals. Lower blood concentrations can be anticipated in BMT patients and those with AIDS, and in patients receiving concomitant treatment with rifampicin. Low concentrations of itraconazole (less than 0.25 mg/l at 4 h) may predict failure of treatment. Levels should be measured in patients with life-threatening fungal infections, in patients in whom poor absorption or drug interactions are anticipated, and when there is treatment failure or relapse. High serum concentrations have not so far been associated with unwanted side-effects.

Serum concentrations should be determined only after the patient has reached the steady state, typically after 1–2 weeks. Blood should be taken just before, and 4 h after, an oral dose of itraconazole. High performance liquid chromatography is the preferred method for determining itraconazole concentrations because microbiological methods detect the active metabolite, hydroxyitraconazole, in addition to the drug itself.

3.13.5 Ketoconazole

As with the other azoles, the results of susceptibility tests with ketoconazole are highly dependent on test conditions. However, provided these are standardized, it is often possible to predict clinical outcome in patients with candidosis. Should treatment failure or relapse occur despite adequate serum concentrations of the drug, the actions described for fluconazole should be taken.

Routine determination of serum concentrations is not required. Low concentrations can be anticipated in patients with AIDS and BMT recipients. Drug concentrations are reduced by concomitant administration of antacids, H2-receptor antagonists, and rifampicin. Low concentrations have been associated with therapeutic failure and it is important to measure the concentration of the drug if this is suspected. The hepatotoxic side-effects of ketoconazole are not associated with high serum concentrations.

4 Dermatophytosis

4.1 Introduction

The term dermatophytosis is used to describe infections of the skin, hair and nails due to a group of related filamentous fungi, the dermatophytes, which are also known as the ringworm fungi.

The clinical presentation of these infections depends on several factors including: (i) the site of infection; (ii) the immunological response of the host; and (iii) the species of infecting fungus. In most forms of dermatophytosis, the fungus is confined to the superficial stratum corneum, nails and hair. However, deeper infection involving the dermis can occur, as in kerion, and this can result in the formation of suppurative lesions.

4.2 The causal organisms and their habitat

There are three genera of dermatophytes, *Trichophyton*, *Microsporum* and *Epidermophyton*. Of the 40 or so species that are recognized at present, some are worldwide in distribution, but others are restricted to particular continents or regions. About 10 species are common causes of human infection.

The dermatophytes are termed geophilic, zoophilic or anthropophilic depending upon whether their normal habitat is the soil, animal or human. Members of all three groups can cause human infection, but their different natural reservoirs have important epidemiological implications in relation to the acquisition, site and spread of human infection.

Although the geophilic group of dermatophytes can cause infection in both animals and humans, their normal habitat is the soil. Members of the anthropophilic and zoophilic groups are thought to have evolved from these and other keratinophilic soil-inhabiting fungi, different species having adapted to different natural hosts. Individual members of the zoophilic group are often associated with a particular animal host, for instance *M. canis* with cats and dogs and *T. verrucosum* with cattle. However, these organisms can also spread to humans.

Those dermatophytes for whom humans are the usual host are termed anthropophilic. These species can be divided into those which are common causes of scalp infections, for instance M. *audouinii* and T. *tonsurans*, and those which cause foot and nail infections, for instance E. *floccosum* and T. *rubrum*.

4.3   Laboratory diagnosis of dermatophytosis

It has been estimated that as much as 50% of suspicious material sampled from infected persons may not contain any fungus. It is important therefore to employ the correct procedures when taking specimens of skin, nails or hair for laboratory investigation (see Chapter 2).

Microscopic examination and culture of clinical specimens should both be attempted on all occasions. If, however, there is insufficient material for both microscopic examination and culture of a specimen, the former should be performed.

The recognition of fungal hyphae and/or arthrospores by direct microscopic examination of clinical material is often sufficient for the diagnosis of a dermatophyte infection, but apart from hair specimens, gives no indication as to the species involved. With hair the size and disposition of the arthrospores can indicate which group of species is involved.

Culture is a more reliable diagnostic procedure than microscopic examination. Because it permits the species of fungus involved to be determined, it can provide information as to the source of the infection and aid the selection of the most appropriate form of treatment. The results of culture can be positive even if microscopic examination is negative, but it is more common for microscopic examination to be positive while culture is negative.

Skin, nail and hair specimens can be cultured on glucose peptone (Sabouraud's) or malt agar supplemented with chloramphenicol to reduce bacterial growth and cyclohex- imide (actidione) to suppress moulds other than dermato- phytes. Most dermatophyte cultures can be identified after 1–2 weeks of incubation at 28–30°C.

It is not unusual to isolate moulds other than dermato- phytes from abnormal skin and nails. In many cases, these are casual, transient contaminants and direct microscopic examination of clinical material is negative. However, certain moulds are capable of causing infection and when this is so, it is important that their significance is recognized. These infections are described in Chapters 6 and 7.

| 4.4 | **Tinea capitis** |
| 4.4.1 | Definition |

The term tinea capitis is used to refer to dermatophyte infections of the scalp and hair.

| 4.4.2 | Geographical distribution |

The condition is worldwide in distribution, but is most prevalent in Africa, Asia and southern and eastern Europe, where it is the most common form of dermatophytosis. Improved standards of hygiene and prompt eradication of sporadic infection have led to a marked decline in the incidence of tinea capitis in North America and western Europe. Favus used to be worldwide in distribution, but is now confined to North Africa, the Middle East and parts of southern and eastern Europe.

| 4.4.3 | Causal organisms |

Tinea capitis is caused by a number of *Trichophyton* and *Microsporum* species. *M. canis* is a frequent cause of the condition in western Europe, but *T. violaceum* is predominant in eastern and southern Europe and North Africa. *T. tonsurans* is predominant in North America, and is becoming more common in the UK.

Tinea capitis due to anthropophilic *Microsporum* species is a contagious disease endemic in many countries. It is primarily a disease of children, being more common in males than females, and most prevalent between 6 and 10 years of age. The disease seldom persists beyond the age of 16. Large outbreaks often occur in schools or other places where children are congregated. The zoophilic *Microsporum* and *Trichophyton* species are seldom responsible for more than minor outbreaks of human infection. Household pets, such as dogs and cats, are a common source of infection, but feral cats are another prolific source of *M. canis*.

Tinea capitis due to anthropophilic *Trichophyton* species

is another contagious disease. It is most common in male children under the age of 12.

T. schoenleinii is considered to be the sole aetiological agent of favus, although infections with other dermatophytes, such as *M. gypseum*, *T. verrucosum* and *T. violaceum*, can sometimes produce somewhat similar lesions. Although *T. schoenleinii* is an anthropophilic dermatophyte, favus is less contagious than other forms of tinea capitis due to *Microsporum* or other *Trichophyton* species. It is usually contracted in childhood and may persist into adult life. Debilitated or malnourished children, or children suffering from a chronic disease such as tuberculosis, are more susceptible to this infection. Instances have been reported in which several generations of the same family were affected.

4.4.4 Clinical manifestations

The clinical manifestations of tinea capitis are varied and can range from mild scaling lesions (similar to sebhorrhoeic dermatitis), to widespread alopecia, or less commonly, to a highly inflammatory suppurating lesion termed a kerion. The latter condition is usually caused by infection with a zoophilic dermatophyte.

M. canis and *M. equinum* (both acquired from infected animals), and *M. audouinii* and *M. ferrugineum* (both acquired from infected humans) invade the scalp hair in a distinctive manner. The lesions consist of one or more discrete, round or oval, erythematous patches of scaling and hair loss (2–6 cm in diameter). These may extend with time to involve the entire scalp. The hairs in these lesions are all parasitized and most of them are broken about 2–3 mm above the surface of the scalp. The hair surface is covered with a dense mass of small (2–3 µm diameter) arthrospores. Infected hairs show green fluorescence under Wood's light.

T. mentagophytes and *T. verrucosum* infections of the scalp are acquired from infected animals. The typical lesions are single and are erythematous and pustular. Kerion formation is common. Infected hairs are covered with chains of large spores and do not fluoresce under Wood's light.

T. tonsurans, *T. violaceum* and *T. soudanense* infections are acquired from infected humans. The typical lesions are erythematous, irregular patches of scaling (0.5–1.0 cm in diameter). The lesions are not well demarcated. The affected hairs often break off at the scalp surface, leading to alopecia and giving a black-dot appearance in dark-haired patients. Other hairs are broken off 1–2 mm from the scalp surface and are often obscured under a layer of scales. Infected hairs are filled with arthrospores and do not fluoresce under Wood's light.

The main clinical manifestations of favus are the formation of crusted, inflamed patches on the scalp, with permanent hair loss due to follicular scarring. The scalp itches and gives off a foetid odour. The crusts (scutula) develop around the follicular openings and can fuse to cover large areas of the scalp. Long-standing favus can lead to permanent diffuse patches of alopecia. Although infected, the hairs tend not to break off, and can grow to normal length. Infected hairs give off a dull green fluorescence under Wood's light.

4.4.5 Differential diagnosis

Tinea capitis is often difficult to distinguish from other causes of scaling (such as psoriasis and seborrhoeic dermatitis) or hair loss (such as alopecia areata and discoid lupus erythematosus). For this reason, Wood's light examination and laboratory tests should be performed in any patient with scaling scalp lesions or hair loss of undetermined origin.

4.4.6 Essential investigations and their interpretation

Specimens from the scalp should include hair roots, the contents of plugged follicles and skin scales. Except for favus, the distal portion of infected hair seldom contains any fungus. For this reason, cut hairs without roots are unsuitable for mycological investigation. One method which is useful for collecting material from the scalp is hair brush sampling.

Direct microscopic examination of infected material should reveal arthrospores of the fungus located outside (ectothrix) or inside (endothrix) the affected hair. The arthrospores can be either small (2–4 µm in diameter) or large (up to 10 µm in diameter) in size. Skin scales will contain hyphae and arthrospores.

In *T. schoenleinii* infection (favus), loose chains of

arthrospores and air spaces are seen within the affected hairs. The scutulum (crust) consists of mycelium, neutrophils and epidermal cells.

Isolation of the aetiological agent in culture will permit the species of fungus involved to be determined. This will provide information as to the source of the infection and aid the selection of appropriate treatment.

Hairs infected with *M. audouinii* and *M. canis* produce a brilliant green fluorescence under Wood's light in a darkened room. However, in recent infections, or at the spreading margin of lesions, the fluorescent part of the hair may not yet have emerged from the follicle and fluorescence can only be detected after the hair is plucked. *T. schoenleinii* causes a pale dull green fluorescence of infected hair. The fluorescent hairs tend to be long, in contrast to the short hair stumps characteristic of *Microsporum* infection.

It is important to remember that creams and ointments applied to scalp lesions, as well as host tissue and exudates, can produce a pale bluish or purplish fluorescence under Wood's light.

4.4.7   **Management**

If possible, specimens for mycological examination should be taken before starting treatment. If oral treatment is being considered, mycological confirmation of the clinical diagnosis is essential before treatment is commenced.

Terbinafine (250 mg/day for 2 weeks) and itraconazole (100 mg/day for 2 weeks) have both proved effective in the oral treatment of tinea capitis, but neither compound is licensed for this indication at present. The duration of griseofulvin treatment depends on the nature of the infection and the clinical response; some infections can take up to 3 months to clear. The usual dosage is 10 mg/kg and this should be given after food. Mycological tests should be repeated 1 month after starting treatment and again before discontinuing the drug.

Various topical imidazole preparations can be used to treat localized scalp lesions, including clotrimazole, miconazole and sulconazole. These drugs are safe and side-effects after local application are uncommon.

To prevent epidemics of anthropophilic tinea capitis due to *M. audouinii* from developing, all contacts of infected children should be examined with Wood's light. Contacts of children with *T. tonsurans* infection can be screened using the hair brush sampling method. It is seldom practical to exclude infected children from school, in view of the long duration of treatment.

4.5 Tinea corporis
4.5.1 Definition
The term tinea corporis is used to refer to dermatophyte infections of the trunk, legs and arms, but excluding the groin, hands and feet.

4.5.2 Geographical distribution
The condition is worldwide in distribution, but is most prevalent in tropical and subtropical regions.

4.5.3 Causal organisms
Tinea corporis is caused by *E. floccosum* and many species of *Trichophyton* and *Microsporum*. Infection with anthropophilic species, such as *E. floccosum* or *T. rubrum* often follows autoinoculation from another infected body site, such as the feet. Tinea corporis caused by *T. tonsurans* is sometimes seen in children with tinea capitis and their close contacts.

Tinea corporis commonly occurs following contact with infected household pets or farm animals, but occasional cases result from contact with wild mammals or contaminated soil. *M. canis* is a frequent cause of human infection, and *T. verrucosum* infection is common in rural areas. Tinea corporis is more common among individuals in regular contact with animals or with the soil. Human-to-human spread of infection with geophilic or zoophilic species is unusual.

4.5.4 Clinical manifestations
Tinea corporis may affect any body site, but is more likely to occur on exposed parts. Patients may complain of mild pruritus. The clinical manifestations are variable, depending on the species of fungus involved and the extent of progression, but in typical cases, round scaling lesions which are dry, erythematous and clearly circumscribed, are seen. The fungus is more active at the margin of the lesions and hence this is more erythematous than the middle, which tends to heal earlier. As the first ring of advancing infection con-

tinues to spread outwards, it may become surrounded by one or more concentric rings or arcuate patterns. Adjacent lesions may fuse producing gyrate patterns. In some instances, particularly when a zoophilic dermatophyte is involved, the lesion may be markedly inflamed and even pustular. The lesions are often more extensive in immunosuppressed individuals.

Patients with tinea corporis often have coexistent dermatophytosis of the scalp, beard or nails. In these cases, the smooth skin infection may be the primary site, or it may have been derived from lesions elsewhere.

4.5.5 Differential diagnosis

Tinea corporis can be difficult to distinguish from other causes of erythematous, scaling skin lesions, such as contact dermatitis, eczema, pityriasis rosea and psoriasis. For this reason, laboratory tests should be performed in any patient with skin lesions of undetermined origin.

4.5.6 Essential investigations and their interpretation

Material for mycological investigation should be collected from the raised border of the lesion by scraping outwards with a blunt scalpel held perpendicular to the skin. If vesicles are present, the entire top should be submitted for examination.

Direct microscopic examination of infected material should reveal the branching hyphae characteristic of a dermatophyte infection.

Isolation of the aetiological agent in culture will permit the species of fungus involved to be determined. This will provide information as to the source of the infection and aid the selection of appropriate treatment.

4.5.7 Management

Topical antifungal preparations are the treatment of choice for localized lesions. Four imidazoles (clotrimazole, econazole, miconazole and sulconazole) and two allylamine compounds (naftifine and terbinafine) are available in a number of topical formulations. All give similar high cure rates (70–100%) and side-effects are uncommon. These drugs should be applied morning and evening for 2–4 weeks. Treatment should be continued for at least 1 week after the lesions have cleared and the medication should be applied at least 3 cm beyond the advancing margin of the lesion.

If the lesions are extensive or the patient fails to respond to topical preparations, oral treatment is usually indicated. Itraconazole (100 mg/day for 2 weeks) and terbinafine (250 mg/day for 2–4 weeks) have proved more effective than griseofulvin (10 mg/kg per day for 4 weeks).

4.6 Tinea cruris

4.6.1 Definition

The term tinea cruris is used to refer to dermatophyte infections of the groin and pubic region.

4.6.2 Geographical distribution

The condition is worldwide in distribution.

4.6.3 Causal organisms

The dermatophytes most often encountered in tinea cruris are *E. floccosum* and *T. rubrum*. Maceration and occlusion of the skin in the groin give rise to warm moist conditions that favour the development of the infection.

Tinea cruris is a common form of dermatophytosis. It is more prevalent in men than women. It usually occurs between the ages of 18 and 60, but is most prevalent between the ages of 18 and 25, and between 40 and 50. Tinea cruris is often acquired from another infected area of the same individual. Autoinoculation from infected feet via towels is not uncommon.

Tinea of the groin is a highly contagious condition and minor epidemics often occur in schools and other communities. The infection is usually transmitted via contaminated towels or the floors of bathrooms, showers or hotel bedrooms, etc.

4.6.4 Clinical manifestations

Tinea cruris usually presents as one or more rapidly spreading, erythematous lesions with central clearing on the inside of the thighs. The lesions, which tend to coalesce, have a raised erythematous border which encloses a brown area of scaling. Patients often complain of intense pruritus. Scratching may result in small satellite lesions which sometimes fuse with the primary lesion altering its outline.

The infection may spread from the inside of the thigh to the scrotum, penis, natal cleft, gluteal folds as well as to the anterior and posterior aspects of the thighs. Localized scrotal infection is quite common: the clinical signs are often inconspicuous.

Tinea of the groin may also spread to other skin folds, particularly to the axillae, which may also be the primary site of infection. Interdigital infection of the hands or feet may also develop secondarily from the groin infection. Infection of the toe clefts may precede the development of tinea cruris.

4.6.5 Differential diagnosis

Tinea cruris can be difficult to distinguish from other causes of erythematous groin lesions, such as bacterial and candidal intertrigo, erythrasma, psoriasis and sebhorrhoeic dermatitis. For this reason, laboratory tests should be performed in any patient with groin lesions of undetermined origin.

4.6.6 Essential investigations and their interpretation

Direct microscopic examination of infected material should reveal the branching hyphae characteristic of a dermatophyte infection. Isolation of the aetiological agent in culture will permit the species of fungus involved to be determined.

4.6.7 Management

Most patients with tinea cruris will respond to local antifungal treatment within 2–4 weeks. Topical imidazoles, such as clotrimazole, econazole, miconazole or sulconazole, and allylamines, such as naftifine or terbinafine, should be applied morning and evening for at least 2 weeks. To prevent relapse, treatment should be continued for at least 1 week after the lesions have cleared.

If a patient has extensive lesions, or fails to respond to topical treatment, or has tinea pedis as well, oral treatment should be given. Itraconazole (100 mg/day for 2 weeks) and terbinafine (250 mg/day for 2–4 weeks) have proved more effective than griseofulvin (10 mg/kg per day for 2–6 weeks).

To prevent reinfection following treatment, the patient should be advised to dry the groin thoroughly after bathing and to use separate towels to dry the groin and the rest of their body. The feet should be examined and treated if tinea pedis is present. Occlusive or synthetic garments should be avoided. If the patient is obese, weight loss may be of benefit by reducing chafing and sweating.

Tinea cruris recurs in about 20–25% of patients. If this happens, patients should be given further antifungal treatment and advice about non-pharmacological control measures should be repeated.

4.7 Tinea pedis

4.7.1 Definition

The term tinea pedis is used to refer to dermatophyte infections of the feet. These infections often involve the interdigital spaces, but chronic diffuse desquamation can affect the entire sole.

4.7.2 Geographical distribution

The condition is worldwide in distribution.

4.7.3 Causal organisms

The anthropophilic dermatophytes *E. floccosum*, *T. mentagrophytes* var. *interdigitale* and *T. rubrum* are the commonest causes of tinea pedis in the UK and North America. *T. rubrum* is the principal cause of chronic tinea pedis. *T. mentagrophytes* usually causes more inflammatory lesions.

Tinea pedis is a very widespread condition that appears to be increasing in prevalence. It often begins in late childhood or young adult life and is most common between the ages of 20 and 50. Men are more frequently affected than women.

The infection is usually acquired by walking barefoot on contaminated floors. Hyphae and arthrospores of the causal dermatophytes can survive for long periods (> 12 months) in human skin scales. Excessive sweating and occlusive footwear are factors that favour the development of tinea pedis.

4.7.4 Clinical manifestations

Tinea pedis may be unilateral, but bilateral involvement is more common. Three clinical forms may be distinguished: acute or chronic interdigital infection; chronic hyperkeratotic (moccasin or dry type) infection; vesicular (inflammatory) infection. A combined clinical presentation may also occur.

Acute or chronic interdigital infection is the most common form of tinea pedis and is characterized by itching, peeling, maceration and fissuring of the toe webs. The skin beneath the whitish build-up of debris may appear red and weeping. A foul odour is sometimes present. The cleft between the fourth and fifth toes is most often involved, but the infection may spread to adjacent areas of the feet, including the toenails. In a patient with supposed chronic tinea pedis, an absence of nail involvement makes the diagnosis of dermatophytosis questionable.

Chronic hyperkeratotic infection is characterized by areas of pink skin covered with fine white scaling. Vesicles and pustules are absent. Hyperkeratosis is usually limited to the heels, soles and lateral borders of the feet. The distribution of the infection may be patchy or involve the entire weight-bearing surface, in which case the disease is termed 'moccasin' or 'dry type' tinea pedis. The condition may be asymptomatic.

Vesicular infection is characterized by the development of vesicles, usually beginning on the sole, the instep and the interdigital clefts. The eruptions vary in size, may be isolated or coalesce into vesicles or bullae, and are initially filled with a clear fluid. After rupturing, the lesions dry, leaving a ragged ring-like border. The disease may resolve without treatment, but often recurs.

In certain parts of the world, concomitant mould, candidal and/or bacterial infection is relatively common in patients with tinea pedis. These conditions usually represent secondary infection following fissuring or maceration of a toe cleft. The secondary infection may induce inflammation and further maceration.

4.7.5   **Differential diagnosis**

The symptoms and clinical signs of tinea pedis can be difficult to distinguish from those of a number of other infectious causes of toe web intertrigo, such as bacterial or candidal infection. Non-infectious conditions which resemble tinea pedis include contact dermatitis, eczema and psoriasis.

Candidosis most often presents as mild interdigital erosion and maceration. It sometimes occurs in patients with diabetes mellitus and is more common in hot climates. It often occurs in conjunction with a dermatophyte infection. Other moulds which produce lesions indistinguishable from tinea pedis include *Scytalidium dimidiatum* (*Hendersonula toruloidea*) and *Scytalidium hyalinum* (see Chapter 6).

Bacterial infection tends to produce more inflammatory lesions, often with marked erosion of the skin. Erythrasma (*Corynebacterium minutissimum* infection) is also difficult to distinguish from interdigital tinea pedis.

Laboratory tests should be performed in any patient with foot lesions of undetermined origin.

| 4.7.6 | **Essential investigations and their interpretation** |

Direct microscopic examination of infected material should confirm a clinical diagnosis of dermatophyte infection. It is sometimes possible to distinguish a yeast infection from tinea pedis. Isolation of the aetiological agent in culture will permit the species of fungus involved to be determined. Media containing cycloheximide (actidione) should not be used if infection with a *Scytalidium* species is suspected.

Wood's light examination of the lesion should be performed to establish whether the patient has erythrasma. The coral red fluorescence characteristic of this condition, does not, however, exclude coexistent tinea pedis.

| 4.7.7 | **Management** |

Tinea pedis will often respond to topical treatment with an imidazole compound, such as clotrimazole, econazole, miconazole or sulconazole, or an allylamine, such as naftifine or terbinafine. Terbinafine should be applied to the toe clefts and other affected sites morning and evening for at least 2 weeks. Imidazoles often need to be applied for up to 4 weeks. The patient may also benefit by applying the cream to the soles to help prevent the infection from spreading. The recurrence rate following topical treatment is quite high, and chronic infection with minor scaling that persists despite treatment is not uncommon. Exacerbations of previous infection may also occur.

Mixed fungal and bacterial infections of the feet are common. For this reason, topical antifungal preparations that are effective against dermatophytosis and candidosis, and which possess some antibacterial action (such as miconazole) are often recommended.

If the disease is extensive, involving the sole and dorsum

of the foot, or there is acute inflammation, oral treatment with terbinafine (250 mg/day for 2–6 weeks) or itraconazole (100 mg/day for 4 weeks) should be given in addition to topical treatment (which should be continued for 8 weeks or longer). However, relapse is common.

Chronic tinea pedis is often associated with nail infection. Inadequate treatment of onychomycosis may result in reinfection of the feet.

Tinea pedis is a chronic condition which seldom resolves if left untreated. Exacerbations, which tend to occur in the summer, alternate with partial remissions. Nevertheless, the prognosis in general remains benign.

It is important to inform the patient of measures that may help to control or prevent the infection. Daily bathing of the feet, followed by careful drying of the toes and interdigital spaces, is important. The patient should also be advised to avoid heavy occlusive footwear, which may increase sweating, and to wear soft absorbent socks.

Once the clinical symptoms have cleared, use of an antifungal foot powder on the feet and inside footwear may prevent reinfection.

4.8 Tinea manuum
4.8.1 Definition
The term tinea manuum is used to refer to dermatophyte infections of one or both hands.

4.8.2 Geographical distribution
The condition is worldwide in distribution.

4.8.3 Causal organisms
The anthropophilic dermatophytes *E. floccosum*, *T. mentagrophytes* var. *interdigitale* and *T. rubrum* are the most common causes of tinea manuum. Less commonly, the condition is caused by zoophilic dermatophytes, such as *M. canis* and *T. verrucosum*, or geophilic dermatophytes, such as *M. gypseum*.

Hand infection may be acquired as a result of contact with another person, with an animal, or with soil, either through direct contact, or via a contaminated object such as a towel or gardening tool. Autoinoculation from another site of infection can also occur. Manual work, profuse

sweating and existing inflammatory conditions, such as contact eczema, are predisposing factors.

4.8.4

Clinical manifestations

Tinea manuum is usually unilateral, the right hand being more commonly affected.

Lesions on the dorsum of the hand or in the interdigital spaces appear similar to those of tinea corporis. They have a distinct margin and central clearing may occur.

Two clinical forms of palmar infection may be distinguished: the dyshidrotic or eczematoid form; and the hyperkeratotic form. In the former condition, periods of partial remission intervene between successive exacerbations. In contrast, the hyperkeratotic form is chronic and spontaneous healing does not occur. It is not unusual for one form to turn into the other.

The dyshidrotic form of tinea manuum is characterized in the acute stage by vesicles which tend to appear in an annular or segmental pattern. These are localized to the edges of the hand, to the lateral and palmar aspects of the fingers, or to the palm itself where the vesicles are rather larger, tense, often single, and contain a clear viscous fluid. Removal of the top of the vesicles exposes a pinkish-red weeping surface with fine scaling margins. Pruritus, formication and burning are common symptoms.

The hyperkeratotic form of tinea manuum is a subacute or chronic condition. It begins as a succession of adjacent vesicles which desquamate. This results in a reddened scaling lesion which is round or irregular in outline and enclosed by a thick white squamous margin from which extensions run straight towards the centre. Once the chronic stage is reached, the disease involves most or all of the palm and fingers. The dry hyperkeratosis, with underlying erythema, readily causes fissuring in the palmar creases. The hand has a mealy appearance because of the furfuraceous scales that remain adherent to the horny layer. This is thickened and black in the creases.

4.8.5

Differential diagnosis

Tinea manuum must be distinguished from other forms of dyshidrosis. This condition, whatever its origin, is usually bilateral or even symmetrical. In its typical form, clear

vesicles are grouped on the lateral and volar aspects of the fingers as well as on the palm. There is little or no inflammation of the base. Dyshidrotic eczema is usually bilateral, but mycological examination is often required to distinguish it and other conditions (such as psoriasis, whether pustular or not) from tinea manuum.

4.8.6 **Essential investigations and their interpretation**

Direct microscopic examination of infected material, such as vesicle tops and contents and skin scales, should reveal the branching hyphae characteristic of a dermatophyte infection. Isolation of the aetiological agent in culture will permit the species of fungus involved to be determined.

4.8.7 **Management**

Local treatment with a topical imidazole, such as clotrimazole, econazole, miconazole or sulconazole, or an allylamine, such as naftifine or terbinafine, will often suffice to clear tinea manuum.

In cases that fail to respond to topical treatment, oral terbinafine (250 mg/day for 2–6 weeks), or itraconazole (100 mg/day for 4 weeks) should be prescribed.

4.9 **Tinea unguium**
4.9.1 **Definition**

The term tinea unguium is used to describe dermatophyte infections of the fingernails or toenails.

4.9.2 **Geographical distribution**

The condition is worldwide in distribution.

4.9.3 **Causal organisms**

Fungal infection of the nails (onychomycosis) may be caused by a number of dermatophytes as well as by a number of other moulds (see Chapter 7) and *Candida* species (see Chapter 5). There is wide geographical and racial variation in the causative agents, but in the UK 85–90% of nail infections are due to dermatophytes and about 5% are due to non-dermatophyte moulds. The dermatophytes most commonly implicated are anthropophilic species, such as *T. mentagrophytes* var. *interdigitale* and *T. rubrum*. Their prevalence differs from one geographical region to another. Zoophilic species, such as *T. erinacei*, are seldom isolated

and usually only from fingernails.

Tinea unguium is most prevalent between the ages of 20 and 50, but the actual incidence of the condition is difficult to assess. This is because many reports do not distinguish between dermatophytosis and other forms of onychomycosis, or between infections of the finger and toenails. It has been estimated that tinea unguium occurs in about 3% of adults in the UK.

4.9.4 Clinical manifestations

Toenails are more commonly infected than fingernails. Tinea unguium of the toenails is usually secondary to tinea pedis, while fingernail infection often follows tinea manuum, tinea capitis or tinea corporis. Tinea unguium may involve a single nail, more than one nail, both finger and toenails, or in exceptional circumstances, all of them. The first and fifth toenails are more frequently affected, probably because footwear causes more damage to these nails. Fingernail infections are usually unilateral.

In cases of dermatophyte nail infection, distal or lateral involvement of the nail plate can progress to total dystrophic onychomycosis. The lesion, which is often white or yellow in colour with irregular edges, appears first at the free end of the nail. It spreads slowly and may eventually affect the entire nail, which becomes thickened, opaque, lustreless and yellow in colour. There is usually some subungual hyperkeratosis which results in the nail becoming detached from the nail bed. The nail plate may crumble, beginning at the free end. Paronychia is seldom present in a dermatophyte infection.

Unusual forms of dermatophyte nail infection may occur in patients with the acquired immune deficiency syndrome. These individuals sometimes develop a condition termed superficial white onychomycosis in which crumbling white lesions appear on the nail surface. This is usually due to *T. mentagrophytes* var. *interdigitale* infection.

4.9.5 Differential diagnosis

The clinical signs of tinea unguium are often difficult to distinguish from those of a number of other infectious causes of nail damage, such as yeast, mould or bacterial infection. Unlike dermatophytosis, candidosis of the nails (see Chapter 5) usually begins in the proximal nail plate and

nail fold infection (paronychia) is also present. Mould infections of nails are described in Chapter 7. Bacterial infection, particularly when due to *Pseudomonas aeruginosa*, tends to result in green or black discoloration of nails. Sometimes bacterial infection can coexist with fungal infection and may require treatment in its own right.

Many other non-infectious conditions can produce nail changes that mimic onychomycosis, but the nail surface does not usually become soft and friable as in a fungal infection. Non-fungal causes of nail dystrophies include onychogryphosis, psoriasis, chronic eczema and lichen planus.

4.9.6 **Essential investigations and their interpretation**

Laboratory confirmation of a clinical diagnosis of tinea unguium should be obtained before starting treatment. This is important for several reasons: to eliminate non-fungal dermatological conditions; to detect mixed infections; and to diagnose patients with less responsive forms of onychomycosis, such as toenail infections due to *T. rubrum*. It is also helpful to repeat cultures after treatment has started to ensure that the infection is responding to treatment.

It is not uncommon to obtain negative results from culture of nail specimens from patients with dermatophytosis. One reason for this is that good specimens are often difficult to obtain. Because dermatophyte infection is a disease of the nail bed, subungual material will often give helpful positive culture results. The following methods are recommended. If distal subungual lesions are present, take scrapings or clippings from under the distal edge of the nail. If there is superficial white onychomycosis, take scrapings from the diseased nail surface. If there is proximal subungual involvement, a nail drill or scalpel may be used to obtain material.

Direct microscopic examination of infected nail material should confirm a clinical diagnosis of fungal infection. It is sometimes possible to distinguish candidal infection, or infection due to moulds such as *Scopulariopsis brevicaulis* from tinea unguium.

Isolation of the aetiological agent in culture will permit the species of dermatophyte involved to be determined. It is essential to inform the laboratory if nail material is suspected of being infected with non-dermatophyte moulds,

so that duplicate plates with and without cycloheximide (actidione) can be inoculated. The results of culture can be positive even if microscopic examination is negative, but it is more common for microscopic examination to be positive while culture is negative.

4.9.7   **Management**

Tinea unguium is a difficult condition to treat. Localized distal nail disease can be treated with topical antifungals, such as amorolfine or tioconazole. Amorolfine should be applied at 1-week intervals, while tioconazole must be applied each morning and evening. Amorolfine treatment must be continued for at least 6 months for success with fingernails and 9–12 months for toenails.

The allylamine terbinafine is now the treatment of choice for patients with dermatophytosis of the fingernails or toenails. Oral treatment with 250 mg/day for between 6 weeks and 3 months is often sufficient to cure a fingernail infection, but toenails may require treatment for 3 months or longer. Treatment with oral terbinafine will also clear associated cutaneous lesions without the need for additional topical treatment.

Itraconazole is another effective treatment for dermatophyte nail infection. This drug persists in nail for at least 6 months and pulsed treatment (in which a week of treatment is alternated with three weeks without treatment) has given encouraging results. Two pulses of treatment with 400 mg/day are recommended for success with fingernails and three pulses of treatment (or more) for toenail infections. Itraconazole is also available for continuous treatment and a dosage of 200 mg/day for 3 months is the most appropriate for severe nail disease.

With griseofulvin, up to 90% of fingernail infections can be cured in 4–8 months, but its low cure rate of 40% in some toenail infections means that it is now less appropriate than terbinafine or itraconazole.

5   Superficial candidosis

5.1   Definition

The term candidosis (candidiasis) is used to refer to infections due to organisms belonging to the genus *Candida*. These opportunist pathogens can cause acute or chronic deep-seated infection in debilitated or immunocompromised individuals (see Chapter 11), but are more often seen causing mucosal, cutaneous or nail infection.

5.2   Geographical distribution

These conditions are worldwide in distribution.

5.3   The causal organisms and their habitat

Although *Candida albicans* is the most important cause of superficial forms of candidosis, at least eight other members of the genus are recognized as human pathogens. Most of these organisms are dimorphic, growing as round or oval yeast cells or as pseudomycelium. *C. albicans* can also form true mycelium, but *C. glabrata* (which used to be classified as *Torulopsis glabrata*) never forms mycelium or pseudomycelium.

These organisms can be isolated from the mouth and intestinal tract of a substantial proportion (30–50%) of the normal population and from the genital tract of up to 20% of normal women. *C. albicans* accounts for 60–80% of isolations from the mouth, and 80–90% from the genital tract. However, it is seldom recovered from the skin of normal individuals, being much less prevalent than other members of the genus, such as *C. parapsilosis* and *C. guilliermondii*. Unlike *C. albicans*, which is seldom found in the environment, *C. tropicalis*, *C. parapsilosis* and a number of other pathogenic members of this large genus can sometimes be recovered from plants or soil.

In most patients, infection is derived from the individual's own endogenous reservoir in the mouth and intestinal tract. In some cases, however, the infection is acquired from another person. For instance, neonatal oral candidosis is more common in infants born of mothers with vaginal candidosis which suggests that infection occurs when the infant takes in some of the vaginal contents during parturition. The hands of mothers and hospital staff are another potential source of infection in infants.

Individuals colonized with *C. albicans* possess numerous complicated and often interdependent mechanisms to prevent the organism from establishing an infection. Efficient protection is believed to involve both humoral and cell-mediated immunological mechanisms. Non-specific mechanisms are also important, but it is well recognized that the contribution of particular elements to protection against mucosal, cutaneous and deep-seated forms of candidosis is different. Even trivial impairments of these mechanisms are often sufficient to allow *C. albicans*, the most pathogenic member of the genus to establish a cutaneous or mucosal infection. More serious impairment of the host can lead to life-threatening deep-seated infection, often with less pathogenic organisms, such as *C. parapsilosis*.

5.4	**Clinical manifestations**
5.4.1	Oral candidosis

Oral candidosis can be classified into a number of distinct clinical forms: acute pseudomembranous candidosis; acute atrophic candidosis; chronic atrophic candidosis; chronic hyperplastic candidosis; and chronic mucocutaneous candidosis (see section 5.4.6).

Acute pseudomembranous candidosis (thrush) tends to occur in infants and in old age. It is otherwise unusual unless the individual is suffering from a serious underlying condition, such as human immunodeficiency virus (HIV) infection or cancer. It can occur in patients using steroid inhalers for asthma or other forms of chronic obstructive lung disease.

Acute pseudomembranous candidosis presents as white raised lesions that appear on the buccal mucosa, gums or tongue. If left untreated, these can develop to form confluent plaques. The lesions are often painless, although mucosal erosion and ulceration may occur. The infection may spread to involve the throat, giving rise to severe dysphagia.

It is important to distinguish this condition from chronic hyperplastic candidosis (oral leucoplakia). The simplest test is to determine whether the white pseudomembrane can be dislodged. If it can, leaving an eroded, erythematous, bleeding surface, then this is diagnostic for acute pseudo-membranous candidosis.

Acute atrophic candidosis usually occurs as a complication of broad-spectrum antibiotic treatment. It can affect any part of the oral mucosa. If the tongue is affected, the dorsum is depapillated, shining and smooth. Tongue movement is restricted and swelling results in trauma to the lateral borders if a natural dentition is present. The mouth is often so tender that the patient finds it difficult to tolerate solid food and consumption of hot or cold liquids causes severe pain.

Chronic atrophic candidosis (denture stomatitis) is the most common form of oral candidosis. It is usually associated with oral prostheses, occurring in up to 60% of denture wearers. It is most prevalent in individuals who do not both remove and sterilize their dentures overnight. The condition is asymptomatic, often being discovered only when a new prosthesis is required. The usual presenting complaint is associated angular cheilitis. Lower dentures are seldom involved. The characteristic presenting signs are chronic erythema and oedema of the portion of the hard palate that comes into contact with upper denture.

Angular cheilitis often develops in association with other forms of oral candidosis, in particular denture stomatitis, but it may occur without signs of other oral disease. The condition is common in patients with moist, deep folds at the corners of their mouth. These angular folds are often due to overclosure of the mouth in individuals who do not wear their dentures on a regular basis or who have old worn dentures. The characteristic presenting signs are soreness, erythema and fissuring at the corners of the mouth.

Chronic hyperplastic candidosis (*Candida* leucoplakia) is an important condition because the lesions can undergo malignant transformation. About 5% of all oral leucoplakias become malignant, but for *Candida* leucoplakias the figure is 15–20%. It remains unclear whether this condition is a hyperplastic lesion superinfected with *C. albicans* or the converse.

The most common site of chronic hyperplastic candidosis is the inside surface of one or both cheeks or, less often, on the tongue. The lesion is usually asymptomatic and the condition is often associated with smoking or local trauma due to dental neglect. Lesions range from small translucent white areas to large dense opaque plaques. Lesions which contain both red erythroplakic and white leucoplakic areas must be regarded with great suspicion as malignant change is often present. In contrast to the pseudomembranous form of oral candidosis, the lesions cannot be rubbed from the surface of the buccal mucosa.

5.4.2   **Vaginal candidosis**

Vaginal candidosis is a common condition, and while most patients respond well to treatment, in some the infection is recurrent and others have persistent symptoms that fail to respond to treatment. Up to 75% of all women will suffer at least one episode of this condition during their lifetime, around half of them suffering a further episode. *C. albicans* is the most important cause of vaginal candidosis, accounting for over 80% of infections. *C. glabrata* is the second most common fungus recovered from the genital tract of women with vaginitis, accounting for about 5% of infections. Infections with *C. glabrata* are apt to be milder, but they should not be ignored as the organism is often resistant to antifungal treatment.

The fact that a certain proportion of women harbour *C. albicans* in the genital tract without symptoms or clinical signs of vulval or vaginal infection suggests that changes in the vaginal environment are required before the fungus can exert its pathological effects. The changes that allow symptomatic vaginal infection with *C. albicans* to occur remain unclear, but the condition has been associated with a number of precipitating factors.

Vaginal candidosis is much more common in pregnant women. Moreover, a significant proportion of women with chronic or recurrent candidosis first present with this infection while pregnant. Vaginal colonization and infection are also more common among women with diabetes mellitus, a disorder which has been implicated as a predisposing factor in other superficial forms of candidosis. Tight, insulating clothing and antibiotic treatment are among the other factors that have been recognized as predisposing to vaginal candidosis. However, aberrations of iron metabolism and oral contraception are no longer regarded as significant precipitating factors.

Most women with vaginal candidosis complain of intense vulval and vaginal pruritus and burning with or without vaginal discharge. The condition is often abrupt in onset and, in women who are not pregnant, it tends to begin during the week before menstruation. Some women complain of recurrent or increasing symptoms preceding each menstrual period. Pruritus is often more intense when the patient is warm in bed, or after a bath. Dysuria and dyspareunia are common.

Vulval erythema with fissuring is the most common clinical finding. This is often localized to the mucocutaneous margins of the vaginal introitus, but it can spread to affect the labia majora. Perineal intertrigo with vesicular or pustular lesions may be present. Vaginitis with discharge is another common clinical finding. The classical sign of florid vaginal candidosis in the pregnant woman is the presence of thick white adherent plaques on the vulval, vaginal or cervical epithelium. This is a useful sign in the non-pregnant patient as well. Often the discharge is thick and white and contains curds, but it can be thin or even purulent. Vulvitis may be present without a concomitant vaginal infection.

Vaginal candidosis is but one of a number of causes of vaginal discharge and must be distinguished from other conditions such as bacterial vaginosis, trichomoniasis, and chlamydial and gonococcal infections. Other causes of mucosal pruritus include herpes infections, contact dermatitis, psoriasis and allergies (including reactions to topical antifungals).

It is important to remember that some patients will have more than one genital infection. Simultaneous infection with *C. albicans* and *Trichomonas vaginalis* is, however, unusual. Candidosis is also less common among women with non-specific genital infection, among contacts of men with non-specific urethritis and among women with bacterial vaginosis.

5.4.3 Penile candidosis

In men, genital candidosis usually presents as a balanitis or balanoposthitis. Patients often complain of soreness or irritation of the glans penis; less commonly there is a subpreputial discharge. Maculopapular lesions with diffuse erythema of the glans penis are often present; on occasion there is oedema and fissuring of the prepuce. Itching, scaling cutaneous lesions are sometimes found on the penis or in the groins.

Men with insulin-dependent diabetes may present with an acute fulminating oedematous form of balanoposthitis with ulceration of the penis and fissuring of the prepuce. White plaques can be found on gentle retraction of the prepuce.

About 20% of male contacts of women with vaginal candidosis complain of soreness and itching of the glans penis soon after intercourse and lasting for 24–48 h. Men who have a penile catheter inserted long term or those using Paul's tubing often develop chronic or recurrent penile candidosis.

The diagnosis should not be made on clinical grounds alone as there are other causes of balanitis and balanoposthitis. Specimens for mycological investigation should be taken from the coronal sulcus and subpreputial sac. Patients should be investigated for diabetes mellitus.

5.4.4 Cutaneous candidosis

C. albicans is the most important cause of cutaneous candidosis. The lesions tend to occur in the folds of the skin, such as the groin and the intergluteal folds, where maceration and occlusion give rise to warm moist conditions. Lesions can also arise in small folds, such as the interdigital spaces between the fingers.

The lesions of superficial cutaneous candidosis (intertrigo) usually develop as vesicles and pustules deep in the groin and other skin folds. Friction leads to rupture of the pustules and development of erythematous lesions with an irregular margin. The main lesion is often surrounded by numerous small papulopustules, termed satellite lesions. Application of topical steroids will alter the appearance of the lesions, making them difficult to distinguish from those of dermatophytosis.

Candida infection of the toe webs is difficult to distinguish from a dermatophyte infection; indeed most cases occur in association with dermatophytosis. Candidosis of the finger webs (sometimes termed erosio interdigitalis blastomycetica) presents as white fissures in the interdigital folds, with surrounding erythema. It is often uncomfortable and may be painful. This condition is not common and is usually seen in individuals whose occupations necessitate frequent immersion of the hands in water and who are also subject to interdigital trauma. Interdigital candidosis is often associated with onychia and paronychia of the same hand.

In infants with the uncommon condition, congenital cutaneous candidosis, discrete vesicopustules, often on an erythematous base, are present at birth or appear soon thereafter. The lesions are most often seen on the face and trunk and may spread rapidly to involve the whole surface in about 24 h. This condition is thought to result from intrauterine or interpartum infection; maternal vaginal candidosis is found in over 50% of cases. The pustules do not persist for very long and desquamate prior to spontaneous resolution of the lesions. In occasional patients congenital cutaneous candidosis can progress to life-threatening deep-seated infection. For this reason, affected infants should be observed in hospital until all cutaneous signs clear.

The precise role of *C. albicans* in the evolution of rashes on the buttocks and in the perianal region of infants, associated with wearing napkins (diapers) remains unclear. This condition should not be considered a primary *Candida* infection as it is preceded by an irritant dermatitis.

Other cutaneous forms of candidosis include the erythematous, macronodular lesions seen in about 10% of neutropenic patients with disseminated deep candidosis, and the purulent follicular and nodular cutaneous lesions seen in heroin abusers (see Chapter 11).

5.4.5 *Candida* nail infection

Candida infection accounts for 5–10% of all cases of onychomycosis. Three forms of infection are recognized: *Candida* paronychia, distal *Candida* nail infection, and chronic mucocutaneous candidosis. Nail and nail fold infections with *Candida* are more common in women than men. Fingernails are more commonly affected than toenails. These infections often occur in individuals whose occupations necessitate repeated immersion of the hands in water and the nails affected tend to be those of the dominant hand. The fourth and fifth fingers are involved less frequently than thumbs and middle fingers. Among the various species implicated, *C. albicans* and *C. parapsilosis* are the most common.

Candida paronychia usually starts in the proximal nail fold, but the lateral margins are sometimes the first site to be affected. The nail fold becomes swollen, erythematous and painful. The swelling is often sufficient to cause cuticular detachment from the nail plate. Nail plate involvement often follows, infection usually commencing in the proximal section. White, green or black marks appear in the proximal and lateral portions of the nail and then in the distal parts. The nail becomes more opaque, and transverse or longitudinal furrowing or pitting occurs. The nail becomes friable and may become detached from its bed. Unlike dermatophyte infections, pressure on and movement of the nail is painful. Bacterial superinfection is common and it is often difficult, if not impossible, to determine which organism is the cause of the nail damage.

Distal *Candida* nail infection presents as onycholysis and subungual hyperkeratosis. It is often difficult to distinguish from dermatophytosis, but the degree of nail damage tends to be less than that seen in dermatophyte infections. Moreover, fingernails are nearly always involved, while 80% of dermatophyte infections affect the toenails. Many patients with distal *Candida* nail infection suffer from Raynaud's phenomenon.

In patients with chronic mucocutaneous candidosis (see below), the organism invades the nail plate from the outset causing gross thickening and hyperkeratosis. This condition is often referred to as total dystrophic onychomycosis.

| 5.4.6 | **Chronic mucocutaneous candidosis** |

The term chronic mucocutaneous candidosis is used to describe a group of uncommon conditions in which individuals with congenital immunological or endocrinological disorders develop persistent or recurrent mucosal, cutaneous or nail infections with *C. albicans*. The disease often appears within the first 3 years of life. The mouth is the first site to be involved, but lesions then appear on the scalp, trunk, hands and feet. The nails and sometimes the whole of the fingertips are affected.

Chronic mucocutaneous candidosis is common in individuals with disorders in which T-lymphocyte activation is impaired or production of T-cell factors needed for macrophage activation is subnormal. These defects are often specific to *C. albicans*, but some patients have more profound defects that involve the T-cell mediated response to other organisms as well. Patients with chronic mucocutaneous candidosis seldom develop deep-seated infection, despite their widespread or generalized cutaneous or mucosal lesions.

Four childhood forms of chronic mucocutaneous candidosis are recognized. Two forms are inherited, one as an autosomal dominant trait and the other as an autosomal recessive trait. The third form is associated with a range of endocrine disorders. The most common is hypoparathyroidism, but hypoadrenalism and hypothyroidism also occur. The fourth form has no recognized inheritance pattern and is not associated with endocrinopathies. In some forms of chronic mucocutaneous candidosis there is an enormous proliferation of epidermal cells which results in disfiguring hyperkeratotic lesions on the mucous membranes, skin and nails.

Adult forms of chronic mucocutaneous candidosis usually occur in association with thymoma or with systemic lupus erythematosus. Like the childhood forms, this disease is characterized by recalcitrant infections of mucous membranes, nails and skin.

5.5 Superficial candidosis in special hosts

Over 80% of HIV-positive individuals develop oral candidosis at some time during their illness. The development of this condition is often the initial clinical manifestation in asymptomatic individuals and is one of several clinical signs that have been associated with an increased likelihood of progression to the acquired immune deficiency syndrome (AIDS). Both pseudomembranous and atrophic forms of oral candidosis occur and although earlier work suggested that the atrophic form, which is often asymptomatic, occurred at higher CD4 counts, this has not been confirmed. The lesions of the pseudomembranous form are persistent and often spread to affect all parts of the mouth. Angular cheilitis has been reported in up to 20% of HIV-positive individuals.

One consequence of the widespread use of fluconazole in HIV-positive individuals with oral candidosis has been a growing number of reports describing the development of resistance to this agent among the C. albicans strains recovered from these patients. In most cases, the individuals concerned had low CD4 counts and were approaching the final stages of their illness. Many had received prior treatment with topical imidazoles or oral ketoconazole and had then been given repeated courses of low-dose treatment with fluconazole.

5.6 **Essential investigations and their interpretation**

The clinical manifestations of oral candidosis are often characteristic, but can be confused with other disorders. For this reason, the diagnosis should be confirmed by demonstration of the various morphological forms of the fungus in smears prepared from swabs or scrapings of lesions and its isolation in culture. As *C. albicans* is a normal commensal in the mouth, its isolation alone cannot be considered diagnostic of infection. Swabs should be moistened with sterile water or saline prior to taking the specimen, or sent to the laboratory in transport medium.

The diagnosis of vaginal candidosis depends on a combination of typical symptoms and signs and the demonstration of the fungus in smears or its isolation in culture. The latter is much more sensitive and reliable (about 90%) than the former (about 40%). Swabs should be taken from discharge in the vagina and from the lateral vaginal wall, and sent to the laboratory in transport medium.

Intertriginous candidosis is often difficult to diagnose if the lesions are other than typical in appearance. Isolation of *C. albicans* from swabs or scrapings is of dubious significance, because the organism is a frequent colonizer of a range of cutaneous lesions. Microscopic demonstration of the organism in scrapings of lesions is much more significant.

The diagnosis of nail fold infections rests in part on the characteristic clinical appearance. However, microscopic examination and culture is needed to confirm the diagnosis. Material can be taken from the swollen periungual nail wall, or from under the nail fold using a disposable microbiological loop or moistened swab. Pus can be obtained from under the nail fold by applying light pressure. Microscopic demonstration or isolation of the fungus from nail can be difficult with proximal lesions, but material from a distal or lateral lesion, together with subungual debris will often reveal the diagnosis.

5.7 **Management**

5.7.1 Oral candidosis

Immunocompetent patients with uncomplicated oral candidosis respond to topical treatment with nystatin, amphotericin B or an imidazole. In infants the infection can be treated with nystatin oral suspension (100 000 units/ml) or amphotericin B oral suspension (100 mg/ml). This should be dropped into the mouth after each feed or at 4–6-h intervals. In most cases the lesions will clear within 2 weeks.

Older children and adults with the acute pseudomembranous form of oral candidosis can be treated with nystatin or amphotericin B oral suspension (1 ml at 6-h intervals for about 2–3 weeks), or miconazole oral gel. The usual adult dose is 10 ml oral gel (250 mg miconazole) at 6-h intervals. It is essential that any medication should be retained in the mouth for as long as possible. Treatment should be continued for at least 48 h after all lesions have cleared and symptoms have disappeared.

Chronic atrophic candidosis should be treated with topical antifungal agents, such as nystatin, amphotericin B or an imidazole. Patients should be instructed to remove and place their dentures in a sterilizing solution overnight. When the condition is resolved, a new prosthesis is usually required.

Angular cheilitis should be treated with a topical antifungal preparation containing a steroid and perhaps an antibacterial agent as well. It is also important to correct the reason for overclosure of the mouth: a replacement denture may be required.

In cancer patients and HIV-positive individuals with oral candidosis the relapse rate with topical antifungal treatment is high and now that safe oral agents are available, these are to be preferred. In addition to antifungal treatment, patients must be given careful instruction in oral hygiene. Denture wearers should remove and sterilize their dentures overnight and smokers should be encouraged to desist.

Oral ketoconazole, at a dose of 200–400 mg/day for 2 weeks, has proved effective in the treatment of oral candidosis in patients with AIDS. Its major disadvantage is that its absorption, which depends on gastric acid secretion, is reduced in achlorhydric patients with AIDS and those taking H2-antagonists, and its metabolism is accelerated in patients on rifampicin (see Chapter 3). Absorption of ketoconazole can be improved if the medication is taken with an acidic drink. Other potential complications are liver damage (albeit rare) and interference with adrenal and testicular steroid synthesis when given in high doses.

Oral fluconazole, at a dose of 100–200 mg/day for 2

weeks, has been found to be more effective than ketoconazole in controlling oropharyngeal candidosis in patients with AIDS. Unlike ketoconazole and itraconazole, absorption of fluconazole is not affected if it is given together with agents that reduce gastric acid secretion. Nor is the reduction in blood levels as marked as that seen when other azole agents are administered with rifampicin.

Oral itraconazole, at a dose of 200–400 mg/day for 2 weeks, is often effective in the treatment of oral candidosis in neutropenic cancer patients and HIV-positive individuals. However, as with ketoconazole, blood levels are reduced when gastric acid production is impaired, and also during concomitant treatment with rifampicin. Administration of the oral solution formulation of itraconazole (200–400 mg/day for 1–2 weeks) has proved successful in patients who failed to respond to the capsule formulation. This may reflect the improved absorption of the solution or an additional topical effect.

Up to 60% of patients with AIDS with oral candidosis will relapse within 3 months of the successful completion of treatment. At present, long-term maintenance treatment is not recommended, because of the effectiveness of azole treatment for acute disease, the potential for drug interactions and for the organism to become resistant, and the cost.

Management of oral candidosis in patients with AIDS from whom fluconazole-resistant strains of C. *albicans* have been isolated is difficult. In the first instance, higher dosages of fluconazole (400–800 mg/day) should be tried, but the benefit is usually transient. If this is unsuccessful, itraconazole can be prescribed, as this has sometimes been found to be effective in patients who had earlier failed to respond to fluconazole. However, it is not unreasonable to expect these patients to need higher than usual doses of itraconazole. Administration of itraconazole oral solution has proved successful in some patients with AIDS with oral candidosis that had failed to respond to fluconazole, ketoconazole, or the capsule formulation of itraconazole. As a last resort, patients with unresponsive oral candidosis can sometimes be managed with parenteral amphotericin B (0.5–0.7 mg/kg per day for 1 week).

5.7.2   Vaginal candidosis

Most patients with vaginal candidosis respond to topical

treatment with nystatin or an imidazole, such as clotrimazole or miconazole. Nystatin requires a longer treatment period and has a lower cure rate than the topical or oral azoles. However, it often useful in women whose condition has failed to respond to azole treatment.

If a patient is to be treated with nystatin, one or two vaginal tablets (100 000 units each) should be inserted high in the vagina at bedtime for 14 consecutive nights, regardless of an intervening menstrual period. If vulvitis is a problem, nystatin cream should also be applied for 2 weeks.

Five imidazole derivatives (clotrimazole, econazole, isoconazole, ketoconazole and miconazole) are available in a number of topical formulations for the treatment of vaginal candidosis. Clotrimazole, econazole, ketoconazole and miconazole are marketed as creams for vulvitis, and clotrimazole, econazole, isoconazole and miconazole are marketed as pessaries. These drugs give higher cure rates than nystatin with shorter courses of treatment and all of them have a similar low relapse rate. These drugs are safe and side-effects after topical application are uncommon. Treatment times range in duration from 1 to 6 nights. Shorter regimens achieve better patient compliance, but treatment courses of less than 6 nights should be reserved for first episodes.

Itraconazole and fluconazole have been licensed for the short-term oral treatment of vaginal candidosis. These drugs are more expensive than topical preparations, but patient compliance is improved. Fluconazole is given as a single 150-mg dose and itraconazole is given as two doses of 200 mg 8 h apart with food.

Women with recurrent vaginal candidosis (more than three episodes within 12 months) present a difficult management problem. These patients often suffer from depression and many develop psychosexual problems as a result of their illness. It is essential to make a correct diagnosis and to ensure that the patient avoids potential precipitating factors, though these may not be obvious. Other diagnoses include herpes infection, allergic reactions, and bacterial vaginosis. Physical examination, investigations to exclude diabetes mellitus, and mycological investigation are essential and, if possible, should be performed when the patient has symptoms but has had no treatment. There is no need to investigate oral or intestinal colonization with *C. albicans* in women with recurrent vaginal candidosis. Trials have demonstrated that oral nystatin treatment, given to reduce intestinal colonization with *C. albicans*, fails to prevent recurrence of symptoms of vaginal infection. The role of sexual transmission in vaginal infection is unknown, and topical or oral treatment of the male partner does not seem to prevent recurrence in the woman. In most cases, symptomatic recurrence is thought to result from vaginal relapse after inadequate treatment of a previous episode.

Many patients with recurrent candidosis can be managed with intermittent prophylactic treatment with a single-dose or multiple doses of topical or oral antifungals given to prevent symptomatic episodes. Local treatment with clotrimazole (500 mg as a single dose) at 2- or 4-week intervals has been shown to suppress symptoms even if mycological cure is not achieved. Intermittent single doses of oral fluconazole (150 mg) are also effective. After symptoms have been suppressed for 3–6 months, regular treatment can be discontinued to allow the patient to be reassessed. Many women do not revert to the previous pattern of frequent recurrence.

Although antifungal drug resistance does sometimes have a role in treatment failure, other factors such as allergic reactions or poor compliance are much more common reasons for a poor response. Nevertheless, drug resistance should be considered if organisms other than *C. albicans* are isolated from women with recurrent candidosis. By comparison with *C. albicans*, isolates of *C. glabrata* are much less sensitive to fluconazole and other azoles. Women with recurrent *C. glabrata* infection can sometimes be managed with nystatin or boric acid treatment.

| 5.7.3 | **Penile candidosis** |

Genital candidosis in men should be treated with saline washes or local applications of an antifungal cream. Nystatin should be applied morning and evening for at least 2 weeks. Clotrimazole, miconazole or econazole creams should be applied morning and evening for at least 1 week. The female contacts should also be investigated. Men who fail to respond to treatment should be investigated for other infectious or non-infectious causes of their condition.

5.7.4 Cutaneous candidosis

Most patients with cutaneous candidosis respond to topical treatment with nystatin, an imidazole, or an allylamine. If the infection is associated with an underlying condition, such as diabetes mellitus, control of the underlying problem is essential. Treatment with combination preparations containing a topical steroid, and perhaps an antibacterial agent as well is often helpful.

In infants, napkin dermatitis with associated *Candida* infection can be treated with combination topical preparations. It is advisable to use preparations containing hydrocortisone, rather than more potent steroids, because of the risk of absorption. Mothers of affected infants should be advised of the basic irritant cause of the problem.

The prognosis in congenital cutaneous candidosis is good and spontaneous cure often occurs after several weeks. The use of topical antifungal agents, such as nystatin or an imidazole, will hasten the cure.

5.7.5 *Candida* nail infection

Topical treatment with an imidazole or terbinafine will often cure *Candida* paronychia when this is confined to the nail folds. The antifungal cream or lotion should be applied morning and evening for up to 6 months. Measures to reduce maceration of the nail folds should be incorporated into the management of such cases. If patients have developed proximal nail damage, then oral antifungal treatment is usually required.

Localized distal nail infection can sometimes be treated with topical amorolfine (applied at 1-week intervals) or 28% tioconazole solution (applied morning and evening).

Severe nail infection seldom responds to topical treatment. In this situation itraconazole is the most appropriate oral treatment: a dose of 200–400 mg/day for 6 weeks or three pulses of 400 mg/day for 1 week per month should be sufficient for most fingernail infections. Terbinafine (250 mg/day) is less effective in *Candida* nail infection than in dermatophytosis and treatment periods of 6–12 months are often required.

5.7.6 Chronic mucocutaneous candidosis

In most patients, oral and cutaneous lesions will respond to short courses of antifungal treatment. Much longer courses of treatment are needed to clear nail infections. However, the improvement is often transient and the infection will recur unless the underlying immunological defect is corrected.

Oral treatment with ketoconazole led to a marked improvement in the condition of a substantial number of patients with chronic mucocutaneous candidosis, but protracted treatment was required to sustain remission and this led to the development of drug resistance in some cases. Itraconazole and fluconazole have now superseded ketoconazole. These drugs are no more effective than the older imidazole, but they are probably safer for long-term use.

6   Other cutaneous fungal infections

6.1   Pityriasis versicolor

6.1.1   Definition

Pityriasis versicolor (tinea versicolor) is a common, mild, but often recurrent infection of the stratum corneum due to the dimorphic fungus *Malassezia furfur*, a lipophilic member of the normal cutaneous flora. The condition presents as patches of fine scaling and hypopigmentation or hyperpigmentation.

6.1.2   Geographical distribution

The disease is worldwide in distribution but is much more prevalent in tropical and subtropical regions, where up to 50% of the population may be affected. In temperate climates, pityriasis versicolor is most common during the hot summer months.

6.1.3   The causal organism and its habitat

The aetiological agent of pityriasis versicolor is a dimorphic, lipophilic fungus named *M. furfur* (synonyms include *Pityrosporum orbiculare* and *P. ovale*). The nomenclature of these organisms is confusing and their classification is still not clearly established. However, recent work suggests that the lipophilic yeasts currently named *M. furfur* (and previously identified as *P. orbiculare* and *P. ovale* according to their microscopic appearance) probably constitute at least four distinct taxa. In this chapter the name *M. furfur* will be used to describe all of these groups.

The normal skin of the head and trunk is colonized by *M. furfur* in late childhood and adult life. Pityriasis versicolor lesions contain a mixture of budding yeast cells, typical of the organism observed in normal skin sites, and numerous small, unbranched hyphal filaments. These filaments, which are thought to be the same organism in its pathogenic phase, are not seen at unaffected skin sites or in culture.

The precise conditions which lead to the development of pityriasis versicolor have not been defined, but host and environmental factors appear to be important. The lesions have a predilection for sites well supplied with sebaceous glands, such as the chest, back and upper arms, and are never found on the soles or palms, which are devoid of these glands. The disease occurs in all age groups, but is most common in adults between the ages of 20 and 40. Instances where non-cohabiting members of the same family have developed the disease suggest a genetic predisposition.

Human to human transmission is possible, either through direct contact or via contaminated clothing or bedding. In practice, however, infection is endogenous in most cases and spread between patients is uncommon. No cases of occupational infection among medical or nursing staff have been described.

6.1.4	**Clinical manifestations**

Pityriasis versicolor is a disfiguring but otherwise harmless condition. The characteristic lesions consist of patches of fine brown scaling, particularly on the upper trunk, neck, upper arms and abdomen. Widespread infection and localized lesions in unusual sites can also occur.

In light-skinned subjects, the affected skin may appear darker than normal. The lesions are light pink in colour but grow darker, turning a pale brown shade. In dark-skinned or tanned individuals, the affected skin loses colour and becomes depigmented. The same patient may have lesions of different shades, the colours depending on the thickness of the scales, the severity of the infection and the inflammatory reaction of the dermis, and in particular the amount of exposure to sunlight, which may vary from one lesion to another.

In most cases the lesions show a pale yellow fluorescence under Wood's light, permitting the extent of the disease to be judged.

6.1.5	**Differential diagnosis**

Hyperpigmented lesions must be distinguished from a number of conditions, including erythrasma, naevi, seborrhoeic dermatitis, pityriasis rosea and tinea corporis. Hypopigmented lesions can be confused with pityriasis alba and vitiligo.

6.1.6   **Essential investigations and their interpretation**

MICROSCOPY

Direct microscopic examination of scrapings from lesions is sufficient to permit the diagnosis of pityriasis versicolor if clusters of round or oval budding cells and short hyphae, which are seldom branched, are seen.

CULTURE

M. furfur cannot be isolated on routine media unless lipid is added. As this organism is part of the normal flora, its isolation does not contribute to diagnosis. To isolate *M. furfur*, scrapings from a lesion can be inoculated onto the surface of a glucose peptone agar plate which is then overlaid with a layer of sterile olive oil and incubated at 32–34°C. Small, cream-yellow colonies should develop within 1 week. Several specialized media are also available.

6.1.7   **Management**

If left untreated pityriasis versicolor will persist for long periods. Most patients respond to topical treatment, but more than 50% relapse within 12 months. Oral treatment is indicated in patients with extensive or recalcitrant lesions.

There are numerous topical agents which can be used to treat pityriasis versicolor. Selenium sulphide (2%) shampoo should be applied at night and washed off the following morning. The treatment should be repeated 1 and 6 weeks later. Ketoconazole shampoo should be applied once daily for 5 days. It should be left in contact with the lesions for 3–5 min before being rinsed off.

Other topical imidazoles, such as bifonazole, clotrimazole, econazole, miconazole and sulconazole, should be applied morning and evening for 4–6 weeks. Topical terbinafine should be applied to the lesions each morning and evening for 2 weeks. Pityriasis versicolor is often a difficult disease to clear and topical preparations may need to be reused at intervals to ensure that the infection is eradicated.

Oral griseofulvin and terbinafine are inactive in patients with pityriasis versicolor. Both ketoconazole (200 mg/day for 1 week) and itraconazole (200 mg/day for 1 week) are effective oral treatments for this condition.

6.2 **Other *Malassezia* infections**

In addition to pityriasis versicolor, two other cutaneous diseases are associated with *M. furfur*. These are *Malassezia* folliculitis and seborrhoeic dermatitis. *M. furfur* has also caused catheter-related sepsis in adults, children and low birth-weight infants receiving parenteral lipid nutrition (see Chapter 27).

6.2.1 *Malassezia* folliculitis

There are three main forms of this condition, in which a cutaneous folliculitis is associated with *M. furfur*. The first, which is most common in young adults, is a folliculitis on the back or upper chest that consists of scattered, itching, follicular papules or pustules. These often appear after sun exposure, or antibiotic or immunosuppressive treatment. These patients do not usually have seborrhoeic dermatitis.

In the second form, which is seen in some patients with seborrhoeic dermatitis, there are numerous small follicular papules over the upper and lower chest and back. The rash is more florid, and is particularly marked on the back. The third form, which is seen in patients with the acquired immune deficiency syndrome (AIDS), consists of multiple pustules on the trunk and face. This form is very similar to the second form, and the patients usually have severe seborrhoeic dermatitis.

Treatment with a topical imidazole or selenium sulphide is often effective, but oral treatment with ketoconazole (200 mg/day for 1–2 weeks) may be required in patients with extensive or recalcitrant lesions. To prevent recurrence, maintenance treatment should be given once or twice per week.

6.2.2 Seborrhoeic dermatitis

This common disease affects 2–5% of the human population, although it is more frequent in men than women. Dandruff is the mildest clinical manifestation.

The role of *M. furfur* in the pathogenesis of seborrhoeic dermatitis remains controversial. However, recent work suggests that these organisms are involved in this condition. In most cases, seborrhoeic dermatitis responds to topical or oral treatment with an imidazole antifungal. Improvement is associated with disappearance of the organisms, and relapse with recolonization. While it is improbable that invasion of the epidermis is responsible for the development of seborrhoeic dermatitis, an indirect disease mechanism such as sensitization is possible.

The lesions take the form of an erythematous rash with scaling and are found on the scalp, face, ears, chest and the upper part of the back. Scaling of the eyelid margins and around the nasal folds is a common presentation. In patients with human immunodeficiency virus (HIV) infection, the onset of seborrhoeic dermatitis is often an early sign of CD4 suppression. Onset may be sudden and the rash is often more extensive than in other individuals.

The clinical signs and distribution of the lesions are typical and mycological investigation is not required.

Topical imidazoles and mild corticosteroid creams are effective in the treatment of seborrhoeic dermatitis. Relapse is common, but retreatment as required is the simplest method of management. Ketoconazole shampoo, used twice per week for 2–4 weeks, is an effective treatment for seborrhoeic dermatitis and dandruff of the scalp. Thereafter it should be used at 1- or 2-week intervals to prevent recurrence.

Oral treatment with ketoconazole (200 mg/day for 1–2 weeks) should be reserved for patients not responding to topical treatment.

6.3 Piedra

The term piedra refers to two uncommon fungal infections in which firm irregular nodules, composed of fungal elements, are formed on and along the hair shafts. These two disorders are distinguished according to the colour of the nodules and the aetiological agent. White piedra is less common than black piedra.

6.4 White piedra
6.4.1 Definition

The term white piedra is used to refer to an uncommon asymptomatic fungal infection of scalp, facial or pubic hair in which soft greyish-white nodules are formed along the hair shafts.

6.4.2 Geographical distribution

The condition is worldwide in distribution, but is more common in tropical and subtropical regions.

6.4.3 The causal organism and its habitat

The disease is caused by *Trichosporon beigelii*, a filamentous yeast that forms arthrospores and blastospores. This organism can also cause deep-seated infection in immunocompromised individuals (see Chapter 27). *T. beigelii* has a widespread natural distribution, being found in soil and water and on plants. It is sometimes carried on the skin or around the anus.

White piedra affects both men and women of all ages, but is most common in young adults. Although there are reports of familial infection, the disease is not particularly contagious. Shared cosmetics or lotions may serve to spread the infection.

6.4.4 Clinical manifestations

The presence of irregular soft white or light brown nodules, about 1.0–1.5 mm in diameter, along the hairs is characteristic of white piedra. The nodules, which are mainly located on the distal half of the hair shaft, are adherent to the hairs but can usually be detached. The uncovered part of the hair shafts and the underlying skin appear unaffected. No broken hairs are seen. The infection is more commonly found on the hairs of the beard and moustache. Less frequently it affects the scalp and genital region. Usually, only localized parts of the scalp are involved. In other sites, however, there is a more widespread distribution of nodules.

6.4.5 Differential diagnosis

White piedra of the genital hair can be confused with pediculosis and trichomycosis axillaris.

6.4.6 Essential investigations and their interpretation

MICROSCOPY

Direct microscopic examination of epilated hairs mounted in potassium hydroxide will reveal that the nodules consist of septate hyphae, arthrospores and blastospores.

CULTURE

Hairs should be inoculated on to the surface of glucose peptone agar plates and incubated at 25–30°C. Identifiable white to cream heaped colonies will appear within 2–3 days. These consist of hyaline mycelium, which is septate and fragmented into rectangular, oval or round arthrospores. Numerous budding blastospores are also present.

6.4.7 Management

Treatment is difficult. Shaving or clipping the hairs of the affected region is usually sufficient to clear the infection, but relapse is common. To help prevent recurrence, an imidazole lotion can be applied to the scalp after shampooing.

6.5 Black piedra

6.5.1 Definition

The term black piedra is used to refer to an uncommon hair disease in which small dark brown to black hard adherent nodules are formed on the distal portion of the scalp hairs.

6.5.2 Geographical distribution

The disease occurs in humid tropical regions of South and Central America, Southeast Asia and Africa.

6.5.3 The causal organism and its habitat

The disease is caused by *Piedraia hortae*, a saprotrophic mould, which penetrates the cuticle, but does not invade the hair shaft itself.

The natural habitat of *P. hortae* other than mammalian hair is not known. Certain hygienic habits, such as the application of plant oils to the scalp hair, seem to predispose to the condition.

Black piedra affects young adults of both sexes with a slight predominance among men. There are reports of epidemics in families and communities. The infection is spread by the common use of combs, hairbrushes or utensils used for washing hair.

6.5.4 Clinical manifestations

The disease is most commonly found on the scalp, but it can also occur at other sites. Affected hairs show from 4 to 8 (or more) firmly attached nodules, 1–2 mm in diameter. These are oval or elongated, hard, dark brown to black in colour, and may surround the hair. The uncovered part of the hair shafts and the underlying skin appear unaffected. Broken hairs are sometimes seen.

6.5.5   **Differential diagnosis**
Black piedra can be confused with trichorrhexis nodosa and trichonodosis, but mycological examination will always confirm the diagnosis.

6.5.6   **Essential investigations and their interpretation**
MICROSCOPY
Direct microscopic examination of the nodules will reveal a packed mass of pigmented mycelial filaments.

CULTURE
Hair fragments should be implanted in the usual media and incubated at room temperature. Identifiable dark brown to black colonies will appear after 2–3 weeks. They have a folded surface with a flat margin. Microscopy of a direct mount reveals thick-walled, septate, branched and pigmented hyphae.

6.5.7   **Management**
Treatment with a topical salicylic acid preparation or an imidazole cream is often effective. However, relapse is common.

6.6   **Tinea nigra**
6.6.1   **Definition**
The term tinea nigra is used to refer to a rare, chronic infection of the stratum corneum due to *Phaeoannellomyces werneckii*, a dematiaceous (brown) mould. This condition often affects the palms. Less commonly it involves the soles.

6.6.2   **Geographical distribution**
The disease has a worldwide distribution, but is more common in tropical and subtropical regions.

6.6.3   **The causal organism and its habitat**
P. werneckii (which used to be named *Exophiala werneckii*) is a saprotrophic mould found in the soil and on decomposing vegetation. Human infection is thought to follow traumatic inoculation.
    Tinea nigra is most common in children and young adults: it has a predilection for individuals who are hyperhidrotic. Although familial infections have been reported, the condition does not appear to be contagious.

6.6.4   **Clinical manifestations**

Tinea nigra occurs most commonly on the palm of the hand. Less frequently, it involves the sole of the foot, or other sites.

The lesion consists of one or several, flat, dark brown to black, non-scaling patches with a well-defined rim. Inflammation is absent. The patches are very small at first, then later expand and become confluent forming polycyclic or irregularly contoured lesions. The pigmentation is irregularly distributed over larger lesions. The disease is asymptomatic and may remain undiagnosed for a long time.

6.6.5   **Differential diagnosis**

Tinea nigra must be differentiated from naevi, from malignant melanoma, and from chemical stains (such as silver nitrate).

6.6.6   **Essential investigations and their interpretation**

MICROSCOPY

Direct microscopic examination of scrapings from the margin of a lesion will reveal rather irregular branched septate brown hyphae.

CULTURE

Scrapings should be inoculated onto glucose peptone agar plates and incubated at 25–28°C. Identifiable olive-black colonies of *P. werneckii* should appear within 1 week.

6.6.7   **Management**

Many methods of treatment have proved effective. Benzoic acid compound ointment or 10% thiabendazole solution should be applied morning and evening for several weeks. Most lesions will disappear within 2–4 weeks, but treatment should be continued for at least 3 weeks to avoid recurrence. Topical imidazoles are also effective.

6.7   ***Scytalidium* infection**

The brown-pigmented mould *Scytalidium dimidiatum* (which used to be named *Hendersonula toruloidea*) is a tropical plant pathogen which can also cause human infection of the palms, soles and nails. More recently, similar infections have been attributed to the related, non-pigmented mould *Scytalidium hyalinum*. In both cases the affected patients have originated from the tropics and subtropics. Unlike dermatophytosis, these mould infections are not contagious.

The clinical signs of *Scytalidium* infection are identical to those of *Trichophyton rubrum* infection. There is scaling of the interdigital spaces, over the soles, and on one or both palms. Itching is minimal. Nail infection may also develop (see Chapter 7).

Direct microscopic examination of scrapings shows fungal hyphae and arthrospores which may be difficult to distinguish from those of a dermatophyte. Both organisms will grow on glucose peptone agar, but are inhibited if cycloheximide (actidione) is incorporated in the medium. Therefore, it is essential to inform the laboratory if skin material is suspected of being infected with *S. dimidiatum* or *S. hyalinum*, so that duplicate plates with and without cycloheximide can be inoculated.

Both moulds are resistant to the modern treatments for cutaneous fungal infection. However, benzoic acid compound ointment can sometimes be used to treat these infections.

7   Mould infections of nails

7.1   **Definition**
The term onychomycosis is used to describe infection of the
nails due to fungi. Nail infections due to dermatophyte fungi
and *Candida* species are described in Chapters 4 and 5. This
chapter deals with infections caused by other less common
non-dermatophyte (mould) fungi.

7.2   **Geographical distribution**
The disease is worldwide in distribution.

7.3   **The causal organisms and their habitat**
Various filamentous fungi other than dermatophytes (see
Chapter 4) have been isolated from abnormal nails. Often,
these are casual, transient contaminants and direct microscopic examination of nail clippings and scrapings is negative. However, certain moulds are capable of causing nail
infection and when this is so it is important that their
significance is recognized.

The incidence of mould infection of the nails is difficult to
assess from published work, but moulds account for about
5% of cases of onychomycosis diagnosed in the UK. Mould
infections of nails have been reported in all age groups, but
are most prevalent in persons over 50 years of age. Men are
more commonly affected than women and toenails are more
frequently involved than fingernails.

There is wide geographical and ethnic variation in the
causative organisms, but *Scopulariopsis brevicaulis*, a
ubiquitous soil fungus, is the most common cause of non-
dermatophyte nail infection in the UK. *Scytalidium dimidiatum* (*Hendersonula toruloidea*) and *Scytalidium hyalinum*
have been isolated from diseased nails as well as from skin
infections of the hand and foot (see Chapter 6) in patients
from the tropics. Other causes of nail infection include
Aspergillus species, *Acremonium* species and *Fusarium* species. Unlike dermatophytosis, these mould infections are not
contagious, but many of them will not respond to the standard treatments for dermatophyte or candida onychomycosis.

104

7.4 **Clinical manifestations**

With the exception of *Scytalidium* species, non-dermato-phyte moulds usually occur as secondary invaders in nails that have previously been diseased or traumatized. This may account for the fact that these infections often affect only one nail. The toenails, especially the big toenail, are more frequently affected than the fingernails.

The disease process usually begins the distal end of the nail or at the lateral margins, generally with a small white superficial lesion, which steadily spreads. The nail becomes lustreless and thickens because of the friable material accumulating on the distal part of the nail bed. The surface of the nail plate becomes irregular and streaked; small pits appear. The colour of the nail also changes; it is white at first but then turns yellow, brown, green or black. The whole of the nail may become friable, or even become detached from the nail bed. There is nothing very specific about the appearance of these lesions.

7.5 **Differential diagnosis**

Mould infections of nails have no specific clinical features. For this reason mycological and histological examinations should be performed on any patient with nail lesions of undetermined origin.

7.6 **Essential investigations and their interpretation**

Laboratory confirmation of a clinical diagnosis of onycho-mycosis must be obtained before treatment is commenced. Methods for collecting nail specimens are as detailed in Chapter 4. It is essential to inform the laboratory if nail material is suspected of being infected with a non-derma-tophyte mould, so that duplicate plates with and without cycloheximide (actidione) can be inoculated.

Isolation of a mould is not a sufficient reason for ascribing a pathogenic role to it without further investigation. Moulds are ubiquitous and their aetiological role must be assessed whenever they are isolated from nail material.

The fungus must be seen on direct microscopic exam-ination and the mould must be isolated in pure culture without the simultaneous appearance of a dermatophyte. It is sometimes possible to distinguish infections with *S. bre-vicaulis* from tinea unguium on microscopic examination:

the characteristic, roughened thick-walled oval spores of this mould are often present in infected nails.

If an opportunistic fungus has been found on mycological investigation, the relationship between it and the nail plate can be determined with the aid of histological sections.

7.7   Management

Mould infections of nails are difficult to treat and even if the mould can be eradicated, this seldom leads to normal nail growth. Localized distal nail disease can sometimes be treated with topical amorolfine or 28% tioconazole nail solution. Amorolfine should be applied at 1-week intervals, while tioconazole must be applied each morning and evening. Amorolfine treatment must be continued for at least 6 months for success with fingernails and 9–12 months for toenails.

Proximal nail disease or severe nail bed involvement seldom responds to topical treatment, even if this is preceded by chemical dissolution of the diseased nail. Nail avulsion can result in permanent damage, but it often leads to some improvement in the appearance of the nail.

There are anecdotal reports that oral treatment with terbinafine (250 mg/day) or itraconazole (200 mg/day) has been effective in some patients with mould infections of nails. However, even if the mould can be eradicated, this seldom leads to normal nail growth.

8   Keratomycosis

8.1   Definition

The term keratomycosis (mycotic keratitis) is used to describe fungal infection of the cornea. This often follows the traumatic implantation of spores into the corneal epithelium, or their inadvertent introduction during surgical procedures, such as corneal transplantation. This infection is difficult to treat and can cause severe visual impairment or blindness.

8.2   Geographical distribution

The condition is worldwide in distribution, but is more common in the tropics, accounting for 30–50% of cases of microbial keratitis in the Indian subcontinent. In temperate climates it is most common in rural districts.

8.3   The causal organisms and their habitat

More than 60 different fungi have been reported to cause corneal infection. Most are widespread in the environment, being found in soil, dust and decomposing plant matter. Their spores are often found in the outside air. Many of these saprotrophic organisms are also common culture contaminants.

Members of the genus *Aspergillus* (in particular *A. fumigatus* and *A. flavus*) are the most common cause of keratomycosis in the Indian subcontinent, but species of *Fusarium* (in particular *F. solani* and *F. oxysporum*) are predominant in many other tropical and subtropical regions. Other causes of keratomycosis include *Candida* species, *Curvularia* species and *Penicillium* species.

Keratomycosis is most common in men, particularly those with an outdoor occupation. It usually follows some form of trauma involving plant or animal matter (such as wood splinters) or other materials (such as metal splinters). The traumatizing agent itself may harbour fungal spores which are thus implanted into the cornea, or the injuring agent may cause a superficial abrasion that exposes the cornea to infection. Seasonal variations in the incidence of the disease

107

have been noted, with infections being more common during the harvesting season in India.

Many patients with keratomycosis have received topical antibiotic or steroid treatment for ocular disease and this is an important predisposing factor. Extended-wear soft contact lenses also appear to be a risk factor for fungal keratitis.

8.4 Clinical manifestations

The clinical manifestations of keratomycosis are similar regardless of the organism involved. The infection is often insidious in onset, with mild symptoms having been present for some time. Often the patient has been treated with antibiotics and the correct diagnosis is not suspected until the condition fails to respond. The most common symptoms include increasing pain, ocular redness, photophobia and blurred vision. Discharge is unusual.

Examination of the affected eye should be carried out using a slit lamp. The usual clinical finding is a raised corneal ulcer with a white, ragged border. Around and beneath the ulcer is a dense infiltrate extending deep into the corneal stroma. Although the lesion has a radiating margin, it is well defined. Discrete satellite lesions often develop. In the more severe cases, involvement of the anterior chamber occurs, leading to formation of a sterile hypopyon. If left untreated, the infection will spread into the anterior chamber and result in corneal perforation and loss of the eye. Enucleation is usually required because of pain.

8.5 Essential investigations and their interpretation

Although the clinical picture is distinctive, the diagnosis of keratomycosis requires the demonstration of fungal elements on microscopic examination of smears prepared from corneal scrapings, together with the isolation and identification of the aetiological agent and the elimination of other causes for the disease.

Because the aetiological agents of keratomycosis are common contaminants of the corneal surface, isolation alone is inadequate for making a diagnosis. Nor is a superficial corneal surface specimen adequate. The organisms are often difficult to find, being located deep inside the corneal stroma, rather than on the surface.

Specimens should be taken using a sterile platinum

spatula to scrape corneal fragments from the margins and base of the ulcer. Swabs are not appropriate. Because the amount of material that can be obtained will be small, it is best transferred to a clean glass slide for microscopic examination and to an agar plate for culture at the bedside. The scrapings should be examined with a potassium hydroxide wet mount or a Gram stain. Some material should also be inoculated on to plates or slopes of glucose peptone agar supplemented with an antibacterial antibiotic, such as chloramphenicol. These should be incubated at 25–30°C (rather than 37°C) for at least 2 weeks before being discarded as negative. The colonies of most aetiological agents of keratomycosis appear within 3–5 days. Isolation of a fungus is more convincing if multiple colonies are obtained on a plate, or if the same organism is recovered on more than one occasion.

If corneal scrapings are negative, but a diagnosis of keratomycosis is still suspected because the patient is not responding to antibacterial treatment, it is essential for the lesion to be biopsied. This should involve partial thickness trephination, with half the specimen being sent for culture and the remainder for histopathological examination.

Anterior chamber paracentesis is not recommended because it is not without risk and the hypopyon, if present, is usually sterile.

8.6   **Management**

The management of keratomycosis entails removal of infected tissue, discontinuation of corticosteroids, and topical or oral treatment with an antifungal drug.

Topical treatment with 5% natamycin solution is often recommended for the initial management of corneal mould infection. Topical amphotericin B remains the preferred treatment for candidal lesions. This drug can be toxic, but a 0.15% solution is well tolerated and shows reasonable ocular penetration. The imidazole compounds clotrimazole, econazole and miconazole are active against many moulds and topical treatment with a 1% solution is well tolerated. Miconazole achieves good concentrations in damaged corneal tissue and the aqueous following topical or sub-conjunctival administration.

Topical treatment should be applied at hourly intervals for the first week. Thereafter it should be applied at similar intervals when the patient is awake. Treatment should be continued for at least 6 weeks for a candidal infection and for up to 12 weeks for a mould infection. Signs of improvement include reduction of pain, disappearance of satellite lesions, decreasing size of the infiltrate and rounding out of the ulcer margin. Negative scrapings during treatment are not significant, and should not be regarded as an indication of response to treatment.

Oral treatment should be considered in patients with severe or worsening lesions. Fluconazole is not effective in mould infections, but shows good corneal penetration. It can be used to treat candidal infection at a dose of 200–800 mg/day. Ketoconazole (400 mg/day) has benefited some patients with mould infection, but itraconazole (200–400 mg/day) has proved more successful.

Surgical intervention is indicated in cases of medical treatment failure. Superficial debridement will improve the penetration of topical antifungal drugs. Superficial or lamellar keratectomy may be effective if the lesion is small and localized, and particularly if it is located in the peripheral cornea. Penetrating keratoplasty should be performed if the ulcer is progressing despite appropriate antifungal treatment.

Fusarium infections often result in rapid corneal sloughing and marked visual loss, and are difficult to treat. *Aspergillus* infections are less difficult to manage with antifungal agents, but the larger the ulcer and the deeper the hypopyon, the greater the likelihood of loss of vision. Even with intensive antifungal treatment, progression to corneal perforation, scleral suppuration or anterior chamber infection can occur. Corneal scarring with consequent reduction in vision is a frequent complication, even with successful treatment.

9 Otomycosis

9.1 Definition

The term otomycosis is used to describe fungal infection of the ear canal.

9.2 Geographical distribution

The condition is worldwide in distribution, but is more common in tropical and subtropical regions.

9.3 The causal organisms and their habitat

Otomycosis is most commonly caused by *Aspergillus* species, particularly *A. fumigatus*, *A. niger*, *A. nidulans* and *A. flavus*, and *Candida* species, particularly *C. albicans* and *C. tropicalis*. Other agents that have been implicated include ubiquitous saprotrophic moulds, such as *Absidia* species, *Acremonium* species, *Penicillium* species, *Scedosporium apiospermum* (*Pseudallescheria boydii*), *Rhizopus* species and *Scopulariopsis brevicaulis*. Many of these moulds are also common culture contaminants.

Otomycosis occurs in adults of all ages and of both sexes; children are less commonly affected. In temperate regions it is most frequently seen during the summer months. It is not a contagious condition.

Otomycosis often develops in individuals with pre-existing aural disease, such as seborrhoeic dermatitis or psoriasis. Bacterial infection is common in such cases, and prolonged use of topical antibiotics and steroids will often result in fungal infection.

9.4 Clinical manifestations

The main symptoms of otomycosis are discomfort and irritation in and around the ear. Sometimes, discharge is present. Obstruction of the meatus can lead to partial hearing loss, tinnitus and giddiness. If, as is often the case, there is concurrent bacterial infection this can cause marked pain and suppuration.

In most cases otoscopic examination reveals that the ear canal is oedematous and erythematous, and is covered with numerous crusts. The drum may appear infected. If *Aspergillus niger* is the causative agent a mat of fungus, often covered with black sporing heads, can be seen. This mass lining the meatus, which it can obstruct, is often described as resembling greyish blotting paper. In chronic infections, eczematoid changes and lichenification of the canal can become marked.

In neutropenic patients, *Aspergillus* infection of the external ear can result in a necrotic otitis externa. There is erythema and superficial ulceration, together with bleeding and discharge. Pain is common. The infection can spread to the middle ear and mastoid.

9.5 Differential diagnosis

The clinical diagnosis of otomycosis is difficult, although a lack of response to topical antibiotics and steroids, and the onset of hearing loss, are suggestive of fungal infection. The diagnosis can be established with confidence only by mycological investigation.

9.6 Essential investigations and their interpretation

Material for mycological investigation should be obtained from the deposits blocking the ear canal. Microscopic examination will reveal branching hyphae, or budding cells or both. In cases of *Aspergillus* infection, the typical sporing heads can sometimes be seen.

Isolation of the aetiological agent in culture will enable the species of the fungus involved to be identified.

9.7 Management

The treatment of otomycosis consists of removal of debris from the ear canal and cleaning, together with the application of an antifungal agent. Topical natamycin or nystatin can be applied morning and evening for 2–3 weeks. Local application of an imidazole cream, such as clotrimazole or econazole nitrate also gives good results. Another method is to insert gauze packs, soaked in amphotericin B, natamycin or an imidazole preparation, for 1 week. These should be replaced at frequent intervals.

10   Aspergillosis

10.1   Definition

The term aspergillosis is used to refer to infections due to moulds belonging to the genus *Aspergillus*. In its most serious form there is widespread growth of the fungus in the lungs and dissemination to other organs often follows. This condition occurs in immunocompromised individuals and is fatal if left untreated. Human disease can also result from non-infectious mechanisms: inhalation of spores of these ubiquitous organisms can cause allergic symptoms in both atopic and non-atopic individuals.

10.2   Geographical distribution

These conditions are worldwide in distribution.

10.3   The causal organisms and their habitat

Moulds of the genus *Aspergillus* are widespread in the environment, being found in the soil, in the air, on plants and on decomposing organic matter. In the home these moulds are often found in dust and on food. Similar contamination also occurs in the hospital environment and can result in outbreaks of nosocomial *Aspergillus* infection. *A. fumigatus* and *A. flavus* are the most common pathogens, but other species, including *A. nidulans*, *A. niger* and *A. terreus*, have also been implicated.

Nosocomial outbreaks of aspergillosis have become a well-recognized complication of construction work in or near hospital units in which neutropenic cancer patients and transplant recipients are housed. In several reported outbreaks, building works adjacent to the unit in which the patients were accommodated led to contamination of the air. In other outbreaks, the ventilation system for the unit drew contaminated air from neighbouring building sites, or otherwise became contaminated.

Lethal invasive forms of aspergillosis have emerged as a major problem in several groups of patients. The first consists of cancer patients and bone marrow transplant (BMT) recipients rendered neutropenic as the result of an underlying malignant disease or its treatment. Most at risk are those patients who remain neutropenic for 2 weeks or longer. Among BMT recipients the use of T-cell depletion and the development of graft-versus-host disease following the transplant are additional factors contributing to the risk of developing aspergillosis. Organ transplant patients are another high-risk group, steroid treatment being an important predisposing factor. Children with the inherited disorder chronic granulomatous disease (CGD) are another group with a high risk of developing aspergillosis: up to 40% of these individuals develop the infection. About 4% of patients with the acquired immune deficiency syndrome (AIDS) develop aspergillosis, the risk being greatest in individuals with late-stage human immunodeficiency virus (HIV) infection.

10.4 Clinical manifestations

Most infections follow inhalation of spores that have been released into the air, and the lungs and paranasal sinuses are the most common initial sites of damage. Infection can also follow the traumatic implantation of spores as in corneal infection (see Chapter 8), or inadvertent inoculation as in endocarditis.

Inhalation of *Aspergillus* spores can give rise to a number of different clinical forms of aspergillosis, depending on the immunological status of the host. In non-compromised individuals, *Aspergillus* can act as a potent allergen or cause localized infection of the lungs or sinuses. In immunocompromised patients, there is widespread growth of the fungus in the lungs or sinuses and dissemination to other organs often follows. This condition is usually fatal, even if diagnosed during life and treated. It must, however, be emphasized that with early diagnosis and treatment, a small but significant number of patients are cured.

10.4.1 Allergic aspergillosis

This is an uncommon condition, most often seen in atopic individuals who develop bronchial allergic reactions (asthma) following inhalation of *Aspergillus* spores. Mucus plugs then form in the bronchi, leading to atelectasis. The illness may be mild, but it is an episodic condition and can often progress to bronchiectasis and fibrosis.

It is thought to result from type I and III, and perhaps type IV, immunological reactions to antigens released from the fungus colonizing the bronchial tree.

The most frequent symptoms include fever, intractable asthma, productive cough, malaise and weight loss. Expectoration of brown eosinophilic mucus plugs containing *Aspergillus* mycelium is common. The radiographic findings range from small, fleeting, unilateral or bilateral infiltrates with ill-defined margins (often in the upper lobes) and hilar or paratracheal lymph node enlargement, to chronic consolidation and lobar contractions.

10.4.2 Fungus ball of the lung

Fungus ball (aspergilloma) formation usually occurs in patients with residual lung cavities following tuberculosis, sarcoidosis, bronchiectasis, pneumoconiosis or ankylosing spondylitis. Haemoptysis is the only serious complication. Fungus balls are usually located in the upper lobes. Less frequently they occur in the apical segments of the lower lobes. Spontaneous lysis has been reported to occur in up to 10% of cases.

Patients are often asymptomatic, but may present with chronic cough, malaise and weight loss. Haemoptysis is the most common symptom, occurring in 50–80% of cases. Most patients have intermittent episodes of small amounts of bleeding, but up to 25% suffer massive life-threatening haemoptysis.

Chest radiographs will reveal a characteristic oval or round mass with a radiolucent halo or crescent of air over the superior aspect. The mass can often be shown to move as the patient changes position. Computed tomographic (CT) scans will help to delineate the lesion.

10.4.3 Chronic necrotizing aspergillosis of the lung

This is an indolent condition seen in middle-aged or older patients with an underlying lung disease, such as inactive tuberculosis, bronchiectasis, sarcoidosis or pneumoconiosis. Many of these patients have other illnesses, such as alcoholism or diabetes mellitus, which can cause mild immunological impairment, or have received long-term, low-dose steroid treatment. Patients with *Aspergillus* fungus balls in their lungs have a similar clinical profile and it is sometimes difficult to distinguish between the two disorders, because chronic necrotizing aspergillosis is often complicated by fungus ball formation.

The most frequent symptoms include fever, productive cough, malaise and weight loss, often lasting for months before diagnosis. The earliest radiological change is a chronic upper lobe infiltrate associated with pleural thickening. Cavitation is common and about 50% of patients then develop single or multiple fungus balls inside the necrotic lung cavities.

10.4.4 Acute invasive aspergillosis of the lung

This form of aspergillosis occurs in immunocompromised individuals and is often fatal, even if diagnosed during life and treated. Those at risk include neutropenic cancer patients, transplant recipients, patients with AIDS and children with CGD. The infection can be further classified as focal or diffuse, the former having the better prognosis. Haematogenous dissemination to distant organs is a frequent complication. In patients with CGD or AIDS a more indolent course is typical and local spread of infection into the ribs or spine can occur.

The most common presentation in the neutropenic patient is an unremitting fever (greater than 38°C) that fails to respond to broad-spectrum antibacterial treatment. Pleuritic chest pain and cough are common presenting symptoms, but haemoptysis is unusual.

CT scans of the chest will often reveal lesions in the lungs of patients with normal radiographs. In neutropenic patients the most distinctive signs of focal *Aspergillus* infection are small nodular lesions that cavitate and larger peripheral lesions. Often there is a characteristic region of lower attenuation (termed a halo sign) around the nodular lesions. Should these cavitate a characteristic crescent of air will appear within the lesions. The signs of diffuse *Aspergillus* infection of the lungs are much less distinctive than those of focal infection and other investigations are required to confirm the diagnosis.

If focal disease is identified on a CT scan or radiograph, percutaneous lung biopsies should be obtained for microbiological and histopathological investigation. Bronchoscopic examination is seldom helpful. However, if diffuse disease is seen on a CT scan or radiograph, bronchoscopic examination is essential. In neutropenic cancer patients and BMT recipients, microscopic examination and culture of bronchoalveolar lavage (BAL) specimens is the most useful method for confirming the diagnosis of aspergillosis.

10.4.5 Tracheobronchitis and obstructing bronchial aspergillosis

Aspergillus tracheobronchitis is most often seen in patients with AIDS and lung transplant recipients. The most frequent symptoms are dyspnoea and wheezing, but some patients develop a cough and fever. The symptoms become more pronounced as the infection develops. Some patients die as a result of occlusion of the trachea or a bronchus, while others develop disseminated *Aspergillus* infection.

CT scans often fail to detect *Aspergillus* tracheobronchitis. Bronchoscopic examination will reveal ulcerative lesions or necrotic pseudomembranes and will permit the diagnosis to be established.

Obstructing bronchial aspergillosis is a non-invasive condition that has been described in patients with AIDS. The presenting symptoms include cough, fever and wheezing. Large mucus plugs full of *Aspergillus* mycelium are expectorated or are encountered during bronchoscopic examination. These plugs form in the bronchi, leading to segmental or lobar atelectasis. Chest radiographs reveal bilateral lower lobe or generalized infiltrates. If left untreated, the disease can become invasive and spread upwards to produce tracheobronchitis. The diagnosis is established at bronchoscopic examination.

10.4.6 Sinusitis

Aspergillus infection is the most common form of fungal sinusitis. Five different patterns of infection can be recognized: (i) allergic sinusitis; (ii) acute invasive sinusitis; (iii) chronic necrotizing sinusitis; (iv) aspergilloma (fungus ball) of the paranasal sinuses; and (v) paranasal *Aspergillus* granuloma.

Allergic *Aspergillus* sinusitis is a recently recognized condition, analogous to allergic aspergillosis of the lungs. The underlying immunological mechanism is not well understood. The disease is seen in patients with an atopic background and presents as intermittent unilateral or bilateral nasal obstruction, with headache, facial pain and malaise. Nasal polyposis may be present.

Acute invasive aspergillosis of the paranasal sinuses is seen in neutropenic cancer patients, BMT recipients, patients with AIDS, and other immunocompromised individuals. *A. fumigatus* and *A. flavus* are the most common aetiological agents. The clinical presentation is similar to that of rhinocerebral mucormycosis (see Chapter 13). The presenting symptoms include fever, nasal discharge, headache and facial pain. Necrotic lesions develop on the hard palate or nasal turbinate, and disfiguring destruction of facial tissue may occur. The infection can spread into the orbit and brain, causing thrombosis and infarction. CT scans can be used to determine the extent of the infection.

Chronic necrotizing aspergillosis of the paranasal sinuses is an ill-defined but slowly progressive condition, analogous to chronic necrotizing infection of the lungs. It can occur in normal individuals, but is more often seen in patients who have received steroids for some other condition or have diabetes mellitus. Alcoholism is another risk factor. Patients present with long-term nasal obstruction and chronic sinusitis. Facial pain and proptosis sometimes occur. CT scans will reveal partial sinus opacification with erosion of the surrounding bone tissue. *A. fumigatus* and *A. flavus* are the usual aetiological agents.

Aspergillus fungus balls are sometimes found in sinus cavities of patients undergoing investigation for chronic sinusitis or nasal obstruction. The symptoms, which include pain, nasal obstruction and headache, are often unilateral. Scans will reveal dense rounded opacities which sometimes contain areas of calcification.

Paranasal *Aspergillus* granuloma formation is most common in the tropics: in East and West Africa, in the Middle East, and in the Indian subcontinent. *A. flavus* is the predominant cause. Affected individuals present with long-standing symptoms of nasal obstruction and unilateral facial discomfort, or with a silent proptosis, but are otherwise normal. If left untreated the infection will spread to the paranasal sinuses, orbit and brain. CT scans can be used to determine the extent of the infection.

10.4.7   Cerebral aspergillosis

It is much more common for cerebral aspergillosis to occur

following haematogenous dissemination of infection from the lungs than for it to result from direct spread from the nasal sinuses. The brain is involved in 10–20% of cases of disseminated aspergillosis, but cerebral infection is seldom diagnosed during life. In BMT recipients *Aspergillus* infection is a common cause of brain abscess. In contrast, in patients with AIDS it is an unusual cause of cerebral infection.

The symptoms of cerebral aspergillosis are gradual in onset. The diagnosis is difficult, but should be suspected in a neutropenic patient who becomes confused, obtunded or somnolent. Multiple brain lesions with infarction due to cerebral arterial thrombosis often result in focal neurological signs, fits and raised cerebrospinal fluid (CSF) pressure.

CT scans are helpful in locating the lesions, but the findings are non-specific. MRI scans will often reveal additional lesions in the brain. Aspiration of material from a suspicious lesion will often permit the aetiological agent to be detected on microscopic examination or isolated in culture. Examination of CSF is seldom helpful.

10.4.8 **Ocular aspergillosis**

Three forms of ocular aspergillosis have been recognized: corneal infection (see Chapter 8), endophthalmitis and orbital infection.

Aspergillus endophthalmitis is an uncommon condition, but it has been described in drug abusers, in patients with endocarditis and in organ transplant recipients. It can arise following ocular trauma or haematogenous spread of the fungus. The latter is more usual in immunocompromised patients. The symptoms include ocular pain and impaired vision. On examination most patients have an iridocyclitis or vitritis in association with yellow–white retinal lesions. Retinal haemorrhage or abscess can occur and hypopyon has also been described. *A. fumigatus* is the usual aetiological agent, but *A. flavus*, *A. niger* and *A. terreus* have also been implicated.

Orbital aspergillosis can develop as an extension from infection of the paranasal sinuses. The presenting symptoms include orbital pain, proptosis and loss of vision. In 25% of cases, the infection spreads into the brain and causes death.

10.4.9 **Endocarditis and myocarditis**

Aspergillus endocarditis is most often seen in patients

undergoing open heart operations, although it has also been described as a complication of parenteral drug abuse. The aortic and mitral valves are the most frequent sites of infection. It often gives rise to large friable vegetations and large emboli are common.

The symptoms and clinical signs are similar to those of bacterial endocarditis. The illness may be abrupt in onset or insidious. Fever, weight loss, fatigue and loss of appetite are common, but non-specific symptoms. Heart murmurs can be detected in 50–90% of patients, and an enlarged spleen in 30%. More specific diagnostic signs include large friable vegetations. Emboli that obstruct major arteries, particularly those of the brain, occur in about 80% of cases.

Myocardial infection with abscess formation or mural vegetations may occur as a result of haematogenous dissemination. Myocarditis has been reported in about 15% of patients dying with disseminated aspergillosis. It can result in non-specific electrocardiogram (ECG) abnormalities or congestive heart failure.

10.4.10 Osteomyelitis

Aspergillus osteomyelitis is an uncommon condition, but children with CGD seem to be at particular risk. In these individuals, spread from an adjacent pulmonary lesion is usual and the ribs and spine are the most common sites of *Aspergillus* infection. In immunocompromised adult patients, the spine is also the most common site of infection, but haematogenous dissemination of the organism may be more common. *Aspergillus* osteomyelitis can also result from the inadvertent inoculation of organisms during surgical procedures.

The clinical and radiological findings in vertebral aspergillosis are similar to those of tuberculosis. Most patients complain of fever and of pain and tenderness at the affected site.

Many patients with *Aspergillus* osteomyelitis also have surrounding soft-tissue involvement, with pleural disease and paraspinal abscesses. Joint involvement is rare.

10.4.11 Cutaneous aspergillosis

Two forms of cutaneous aspergillosis have been described in immunocompromised patients. In the first, the lesion arises at a catheter insertion site in patients who have had contaminated splints applied to their skin. The lesion, which may act as the source of a subsequent disseminated infection, begins as an erythematous to violaceous, indurated plaque and evolves into a necrotic ulcer covered with a black eschar.

In about 5% of patients with invasive aspergillosis, haematogenous spread of infection gives rise to cutaneous lesions. These may be single or multiple, well-circumscribed, maculopapular lesions that become pustular. They evolve into ulcers with distinct borders covered with a black eschar. The lesions enlarge and may become confluent.

10.4.12 Other forms of aspergillosis

Although gastrointestinal tract infection has been detected in 40–50% of patients dying with disseminated aspergillosis, this condition is seldom diagnosed during life. The oesophagus is the most frequent site of involvement, but intestinal ulcers also occur and these often result in bleeding or perforation.

Hepatic and/or splenic infection has been seen in up to 30% of patients with disseminated aspergillosis. The symptoms include liver tenderness, abdominal pain and jaundice, but many patients are asymptomatic. CT scans will reveal numerous, small radiolucent lesions scattered throughout the liver. Modest elevations in alkaline phosphatase or bilirubin concentrations can often be detected.

Renal infection has been detected in 30% of patients dying with disseminated aspergillosis. Symptoms are uncommon and renal function is seldom impaired.

10.5 Aspergillosis in special hosts
10.5.1 Patients with AIDS

Aspergillus infection is an emerging problem in patients with AIDS, developing in up to 4% of these individuals. Most cases have occurred in patients with late- or end-stage disease, with low CD4 counts. The factors which predispose patients with AIDS to aspergillosis are not well understood: neutropenia and previous steroid treatment are accepted risk factors, but the significance of other factors is less clear.

The lung is the most common site of *Aspergillus* infection in patients with AIDS, being involved in more than 70% of cases. Several different patterns of infection have been recognized, including invasive aspergillosis, *Aspergillus* tracheobronchitis and obstructing bronchial aspergillosis. The diagnosis can be difficult to establish, but broncho-scopic examination is often helpful. Cerebral infection has also been reported, but is seldom diagnosed while the patient is alive. The response to antifungal treatment of patients with AIDS with aspergillosis is much poorer than that of other patients. Most patients with AIDS with this infection will die, even with aggressive treatment.

10.6 Essential investigations and their interpretation

Establishing the diagnosis of aspergillosis in a compromised patient is difficult because the clinical presentation is non-specific and because the fungus is seldom isolated from blood or other fluids, or from sputum. Interpretation of serological test results is also difficult because failure to detect precipitins in a compromised individual does not mean that aspergillosis is not present. Nor is the detection of circulating antigen a consistent finding in such patients.

10.6.1 Microscopy

Direct microscopic examination of sputum preparations is often helpful in the diagnosis of allergic aspergillosis, because abundant septate mycelium with characteristic dichotomous branching is usually seen.

Microscopic examination of sputum is seldom helpful in patients with suspected invasive aspergillosis, but exam-ination of BAL fluid specimens is often rewarding. Typical mycelium may also be detected in wet preparations of necrotic material from cutaneous lesions or sinus washings, but isolation of the aetiological agent in culture is essential to confirm the diagnosis.

The most reliable method for the diagnosis of acute invasive aspergillosis is the examination of stained tissue sections. The detection of non-pigmented, septate filaments which show repeated dichotomous branching is character-istic of *Aspergillus* infection. However, other less common organisms, such as *Fusarium* species and *Scedosporium apiospermum* (*Pseudallescheria boydii*), appear similar. More precise identification can sometimes be achieved with immunochemical staining methods.

10.6.2   **Culture**
The definitive diagnosis of aspergillosis depends upon the isolation of the aetiological agent in culture. The fungus may be recovered from sputum specimens from patients with allergic aspergillosis, but cultures from patients with other forms of aspergillosis are less successful. Moreover, because *Aspergillus* species are commonly found in the air, their isolation must be interpreted with caution. Their isolation from sputum is more convincing if multiple colonies are obtained on a plate or the same fungus is recovered on more than one occasion.

If sputum cannot be obtained from an immunocompromised patient with a pulmonary infiltrate, BAL specimens should be obtained. Isolation of an *Aspergillus* species from such specimens is often indicative of infection, but the success rate does depend on the patient group and the pattern of disease. In neutropenic cancer patients and BMT recipients with diffuse infection, culture of BAL fluid is positive in up to 60% of cases. The success rate is lower in organ transplant patients, with the exception of lung transplant recipients. Culture of BAL fluid is seldom helpful in patients with focal lung lesions.

Aspergillus species are seldom recovered from blood, urine or CSF specimens, although cultures of the former have been positive in occasional patients with endocarditis. More often, however, their isolation is due to contamination. It has not been established whether lysis-centrifugation is any more useful than traditional blood culture methods in the diagnosis of aspergillosis.

The diagnosis of *Aspergillus* sinusitis is less difficult to establish than infection at other sites. The fungus can usually be isolated from sinus washings or biopsies of the necrotic lesions in the nose or palate.

10.6.3   **Skin tests**
Skin tests with *Aspergillus* antigens are useful in the diagnosis of allergic aspergillosis. Patients with uncomplicated asthma due to *Aspergillus* give an immediate type I reaction. Those with allergic aspergillosis give an immediate type I reaction and 70% also give a delayed type III reaction.

10.6.4   **Serological tests**
Tests for *Aspergillus* precipitins are often helpful in the

diagnosis of the different forms of aspergillosis that occur in the non-compromised patient. Precipitins can be detected in up to 70% of patients with allergic aspergillosis and over 90% of patients with fungus balls in their lung.

The precipitin test is also useful for diagnosing chronic necrotizing aspergillosis of the lung and other invasive forms of *Aspergillus* infection, such as endocarditis, provided the patient is not immunosuppressed.

The detection of precipitins in a neutropenic patient with unresponsive fever or a pulmonary infiltrate is often sufficient to prompt the initiation of antifungal treatment, but it must be stressed that a positive test result is not proof of infection. Nor does a negative precipitin test result preclude the diagnosis of aspergillosis in an immunosuppressed patient, because such individuals are often incapable of mounting a detectable serological response.

Tests for the detection of *Aspergillus* antigen in blood and other biological fluids offer an alternative means of diagnosing aspergillosis in the immunocompromised patient. However, a negative antigen test result does not exclude the diagnosis of aspergillosis, particularly if only a single specimen has been tested and the patient has clinical signs consistent with the infection.

Low concentrations of galactomannan, a cell wall component of *Aspergillus* that appears to be a specific indicator of invasive disease, have been detected in serum and urine specimens from infected patients. However, *Aspergillus* galactomannan is rapidly cleared from the circulation and frequent sampling is essential. Latex particle agglutination (LPA) and enzyme-linked immunoadsorbent assay (ELISA) tests have been marketed for the detection of *Aspergillus* galactomannan (Sanofi Diagnostics Pasteur). Initial reports indicate that ELISA is more sensitive than LPA, detecting galactomannan earlier and giving positive results over longer periods of time.

10.7 Management
10.7.1 Allergic aspergillosis

Mild disease may not require treatment. Prednisone is the drug of choice because it is effective in reducing symptoms, improving chest radiographs, and abolishing positive sputum cultures. The usual dosage regimen is 1.0 mg/kg per day until radiographs are clear, then 0.5 mg/kg per day for 2 weeks. The same dose is then given at 48-h intervals for another 3–6 months, and then the dose is tapered off over another 3 months. The initial regimen should be resumed if the condition recurs. Bronchodilators and postural drainage may help to prevent mucus plugging. Treatment with anti-fungal agents is not thought to be helpful.

10.7.2 Fungus ball of the lung

Surgical removal of the lesion is indicated if massive or recurrent haemoptysis should occur. On occasion, segmental or wedge resection will suffice, but lobectomy is usually required to ensure complete eradication of the disease.

If surgical intervention is contraindicated, endobronchial instillation or percutaneous injection of amphotericin B may be helpful. The optimum dosage has not been determined, but 10–20 mg of amphotericin B in 10–20 ml distilled water instilled two or three times per week for about 6 weeks has proved successful. Larger doses (40–50 mg) have been instilled into lung cavities using percutaneous catheters.

The treatment of mild to moderate bleeding and asymp-tomatic patients remains controversial, but observation without intervention may be the best form of management.

10.7.3 Chronic necrotizing aspergillosis of the lung

Treatment with an antifungal drug, such as itraconazole (200–400 mg/day), will often relieve the symptoms of this condition, but surgical resection of necrotic lung and sur-rounding infiltrated tissue is usually required to eradicate this form of aspergillosis. Medical treatment is often the best option for older patients with a poor prognosis because of other underlying lung disease. In healthier patients con-sideration should be given to both parenteral and local administration of amphotericin B, as well as surgical resection.

10.7.4 Acute invasive aspergillosis of the lung

The successful management of acute invasive aspergillosis in the immunocompromised patient depends on the prompt initiation of antifungal treatment. The response rate differs from one host group to another and depends on the length of time over which treatment is administered. In BMT recipients the response rate is about 10% and in neutropenic cancer patients it is around 30%. Heart and renal transplant patients have a response rate of about 50%, but liver transplant recipients have a rate of 5–10%. Patients who have survived have all received at least 2 weeks of antifungal treatment. In neutropenic patients the prognosis is poor if the neutrophil count does not recover. Limited clinical experience suggests that shortening the duration of neutropenia with colony-stimulating factors may be beneficial in treating the infection.

Amphotericin B is the standard treatment for this form of aspergillosis. There are numerous regimens for administration of this drug, but widespread agreement that in immunocompromised patients it is important to give the full dose of amphotericin B from the outset (see Chapter 3). High doses must be used (at least 1.0 mg/kg).

Administration of one of the lipid-based forms of amphotericin B should be considered in patients who fail to respond to the conventional formulation, or who develop side-effects that necessitate discontinuation of the drug, or in whom the conventional formulation is contraindicated because of renal impairment. There are different dosage recommendations for the various lipid-based preparations (see Chapter 3). It remains unclear as to whether these new formulations differ from each other or the conventional form in terms of clinical benefit in aspergillosis.

Oral treatment with itraconazole has often proved successful in patients with invasive *Aspergillus* infection of the lungs. Success has sometimes been achieved in neutropenic patients who had earlier failed to respond to amphotericin B. The recommended dose of itraconazole is 400 mg/day taken with food, but some clinicians have used loading doses of 600 mg/day at the start of treatment. Absorption of the capsule formulation of the drug from the gastrointestinal tract can be a problem in neutropenic patients and those with AIDS, and blood concentrations should be measured at regular intervals. Higher dosages or substitution of the oral solution formulation should ensure adequate blood levels (see Chapter 3).

The optimum duration of treatment has not been established, but it should be continued for as long as the patient is immunocompromised and until there has been complete or near complete resolution of disease. In neutropenic patients this means continuing treatment until the neutrophil count is greater than $1 \times 10^9/l$ and until relevant radiological abnormalities disappear. This can take weeks or months. Patients with AIDS and organ transplant recipients also require long-term treatment. Clinicians often prefer to change from parenteral amphotericin B treatment to oral itraconazole after the first 2–3 weeks. This is reasonable provided that the patient has no problems with itraconazole absorption.

Prophylactic treatment with itraconazole (400 mg/day) does appear to reduce the incidence of invasive *Aspergillus* infection in neutropenic cancer patients and BMT recipients (see Chapter 3). Absorption of the capsule formulation from the gastrointestinal tract can be a problem, but substitution of the oral solution formulation should ensure adequate blood concentrations. Fluconazole offers no protection against this infection.

The shortcomings of current methods of diagnosis often require clinicians to begin empirical amphotericin B treatment without waiting for formal proof that a neutropenic patient with persistent fever (greater than 72–96 h duration), resistant to antibacterial drugs, has aspergillosis. Empirical treatment should be initiated with the usual test dose (1 mg) of amphotericin B. If possible, the full therapeutic dosage level (1.0 mg/kg of the conventional formulation) should be reached within the first 24 h of treatment. Should the conventional formulation be contraindicated, one of the lipid-based formulations should be used instead.

Neutropenic patients who recover from aspergillosis may suffer from reactivation of the infection during subsequent periods of immunosuppression. One solution to this problem is to begin empirical treatment with amphotericin B (1.0 mg/kg per day of the conventional formulation) not less than 48 h before antileukaemic treatment is commenced. The drug should then be continued until the neutrophil count has recovered.

Some clinicians recommend immediate surgical resection of one or more localized *Aspergillus* lesions in the lungs during neutropenia. Most, however, reserve lung resection for patients with persistent *Aspergillus* infection who require further induction treatment or BMT, for those with significant haemoptysis, or for those with focal lesions in a central location. The latter group are at high risk of death from perforation of a bronchus, the trachea, or one of the great vessels, and rapid surgical intervention is essential.

10.7.5 **Tracheobronchitis and obstructing bronchial aspergillosis**

In patients with AIDS, *Aspergillus* tracheobronchitis can sometimes be controlled with amphotericin B (1.0 mg/kg per day) or itraconazole (400 mg/day). The absorption of itraconazole in late-stage AIDS is often poor, and interactions with other drugs (such as rifampicin) can be a problem. Blood concentrations of itraconazole should be measured at regular intervals.

Patients with obstructing bronchial aspergillosis often respond to oral treatment with itraconazole (400 mg/day).

10.7.6 **Sinusitis**

Allergic *Aspergillus* sinusitis can be treated with prednisolone. The usual dosage regimen is 20–30 mg/day reducing once the symptoms have alleviated.

Immunocompromised patients with acute invasive sinusitis should be treated with amphotericin B (1.0 mg/kg per day). Lipid-based formulations of the drug can be used in patients who develop side-effects, and in those in whom the conventional formulation is contraindicated because of renal impairment. Surgical debridement of infected sinus material is useful, but should not be done during neutropenia because haemorrhage and other complications are frequent.

Treatment of chronic necrotizing aspergillosis of the sinuses consists of surgical debridement, with removal of all necrotic material. Patients should then be given a prolonged course of treatment with itraconazole (400–600 mg/day for 6 months). Surgical debridement is also recommended for patients with an *Aspergillus* fungus ball in the sinuses. It is unusual for this condition to recur provided adequate sinus drainage can be instituted.

In some cases of paranasal *Aspergillus* granuloma, surgical removal of infected material, with drainage and aeration, is curative. Often, however, the condition will recur necessitating further surgical intervention. The long-term results are generally poor. Postoperative treatment with itraconazole (200–400 mg/day for at least 6 weeks) has reduced the relapse rate and is recommended for all patients.

10.7.7   **Cerebral aspergillosis**
This infection has a poor prognosis and even with aggressive treatment, most patients will die. The lesions are often located deep in the brain and are difficult to remove without causing serious damage. Several patients have survived following surgical resection and treatment with high doses of the liposomal formulation of amphotericin B. There are also anecdotal reports of patients who have recovered following treatment with high doses of itraconazole (800 mg/day).

10.7.8   **Endophthalmitis**
Aspergillus endophthalmitis requires both medical and surgical treatment. Intravitreal levels of amphotericin B following parenteral administration are insufficient to treat this infection and intravitreal dosing is required. This will result in inflammation and retinal damage, but doses up to 10 µg can be tolerated. Surgical debridement is an essential part of the management of this infection.

10.7.9   **Endocarditis**
Aspergillus endocarditis requires aggressive medical and surgical treatment. Treatment with amphotericin B (1.0 mg/kg per day) should be commenced as soon as the diagnosis is made. Infected valves should be replaced 1–2 weeks after treatment has started, but earlier surgical intervention is indicated if there are large vegetations, signs of heart failure, or dysfunction of a prosthesis. The optimum length of treatment is uncertain, but 2–3 months has been recommended to reduce the likelihood of relapse.

Treatment with a lipid-based formulation of amphotericin B should be considered in patients who fail to respond to the conventional formulation, or who develop side-effects that necessitate discontinuation of the drug. There is insufficient experience with itraconazole to recommend it as a first-line treatment.

10.7.10   **Osteomyelitis**
Amphotericin B (1.0 mg/kg per day) remains the treatment of choice for patients with *Aspergillus* osteomyelitis, but successful management often requires aggressive surgical debridement of necrotic tissue. Long-term treatment with itraconazole (400 mg/day) has proved successful in some patients.

10.7.11 **Cutaneous aspergillosis**

Amphotericin B (1.0 mg/kg per day) is the treatment of choice for cutaneous aspergillosis. Surgical debridement is essential for successful management of lesions that arise at catheter insertion sites. This should not be done until the neutrophil count has recovered.

11   Deep candidosis

11.1   Definition
The term candidosis (candidiasis) is used to refer to infections due to organisms belonging to the genus *Candida*. In addition to causing mucosal and cutaneous infection (see Chapter 5), these opportunist pathogens can cause acute or chronic deep-seated infection in immunocompromised or debilitated individuals. This may be confined to one organ or become widespread (disseminated candidosis).

11.2   Geographical distribution
These conditions are worldwide in distribution.

11.3   The causal organisms and their habitat
Candida albicans is the predominant cause of both superficial and deep-seated forms of candidosis, although the proportion of serious infections attributed to other members of the genus is rising. There is, however, considerable variation in the range of organisms isolated in different hospitals and different patient groups. In the 1970s *C. tropicalis* emerged as an important pathogen in neutropenic cancer patients and *C. parapsilosis* infection became more common in patients receiving parenteral nutrition. In the 1990s changes in antifungal drug usage have led to a reduction in the number of *C. albicans* and *C. tropicalis* infections in some institutions, and resulted in higher rates of colonization and infection with other organisms, such as *C. glabrata* and *C. krusei*, which are rather less susceptible to antifungal treatment. These changes have highlighted the need for careful speciation of organisms before commencing treatment.

These organisms are found in the mouth and gastrointestinal tract of around 30–50% of normal individuals, but much higher isolation rates have been recorded among patients receiving medical attention. In most cases deep-seated infection is endogenous in origin, but transmission of organisms from person to person can also occur. Outbreaks of candidosis in neonatal and surgical intensive care units

(ICU) have sometimes been attributed to carriage of organisms on the hands of hospital staff.

Lethal, deep-seated forms of candidosis have emerged as a significant problem in several distinct groups of patients. The first consists of individuals rendered neutropenic as the result of an underlying malignant disease or its treatment: the gastrointestinal tract is the principal source of infection in this group and the liver, spleen and lungs are often involved. A second important group consists of surgical and ICU patients (including neonates). These individuals are debilitated, but not neutropenic: disruption of natural anatomical barriers permits the organisms to gain access to the circulation. Patients who have had organ transplants, or operations on the heart, lungs or gastrointestinal tract are most at risk of developing candidosis. Groups of patients less commonly affected include those receiving total parenteral nutrition, those on peritoneal dialysis or with cerebrospinal fluid (CSF) shunts, and parenteral drug abusers.

The incidence of candidosis has increased since the 1980s. The organisms have become the fourth most common bloodstream pathogens in North American hospitals, accounting for 10% of all bloodstream infections and 25% of all urinary tract infections in the ICU setting.

11.4	**Clinical manifestations**
11.4.1	Oesophagitis

This condition often develops in patients with the acquired immune deficiency syndrome (AIDS) or following treatment for cancer. It tends to occur in patients with oral candidosis, but must be distinguished from cytomegalovirus and herpes simplex virus oesophagitis, which can give rise to similar symptoms and clinical and radiological findings. Up to 30% of patients with AIDS with oesophageal candidosis have concurrent viral oesophagitis.

The principal symptoms are oesophadynia and dysphagia. In patients with more advanced infection, barium contrast radiographs will often reveal irregular ragged mucosal margins, ulcers, large filling defects or oedematous mucosal folds. However, endoscopic examination is required to confirm the cause of the ulceration. The characteristic finding is white plaques with intense inflammation. This method has permitted a diagnosis of oesophageal candidosis to be established in up to 25% of patients with normal oesophagrams.

11.4.2 Gastrointestinal candidosis

Although gastric candidosis is common in debilitated cancer patients, this condition is often asymptomatic and is seldom diagnosed during life. Mucosal ulcerations are the most common lesions, but it is unclear to what extent these are chronic gastric ulcers superinfected with *Candida*. Perforation can lead to disseminated infection.

Intestinal candidosis is a controversial condition. It is clear that intestinal infection does result in mucosal ulceration in some debilitated cancer patients and those with AIDS. It is much more difficult to be certain whether intestinal colonization leads to illness in less sick individuals. It has been claimed that *Candida* colonization can produce an alarming range of symptoms, including weight loss, headaches, diarrhoea and general malaise. However, these claims have not been subjected to rigorous clinical investigation.

11.4.3 Pulmonary candidosis

This condition occurs in debilitated or neutropenic patients, but is seldom diagnosed during life. It can arise following haematogenous dissemination of organisms or as a result of endobronchial inoculation of the lung. In low-birth-weight infants, infection often follows aspiration of organisms from the mouth.

The clinical and radiological presentation is non-specific. Haematogenous dissemination gives rise to diffuse nodular infiltrates affecting both lungs. Aspiration of contaminated oral secretions results in a local or diffuse bronchopneumonia. Lung biopsies are the only reliable means of establishing a diagnosis of candidosis.

11.4.4 CNS candidosis

This is uncommon. Meningitis is sometimes seen in low birth-weight infants with deep-seated candidosis and in neurosurgical patients with ventriculoperitoneal shunts. Infection occurs as a result of haematogenous dissemination or direct inoculation of organisms into the subdural space. It often follows an indolent course with minimal fever.

The diagnosis is difficult, but *Candida* meningitis should

be suspected in a neurosurgical patient with bacterial meningitis who fails to respond or deteriorates despite appropriate antibacterial treatment. It should also be suspected in a patient with other signs of disseminated candidosis who develops neurological signs.

The CSF findings are indistinguishable from those of bacterial meningitis. The protein concentration may be increased, the glucose concentration may be low or normal, and a neutrophilic or lymphocytic pleocytosis may be present. *C. albicans* is the principal aetiological agent.

Other forms of central nervous system (CNS) candidosis include brain abscess and diffuse metastatic encephalitis. These manifestations are seldom diagnosed during life. Large brain abscesses may give rise to focal neurological signs. The lesions can be detected with computed tomographic (CT) or magnetic resonance imaging (MRI) scans. More often, however, haematogenous spread of organisms results in multiple small lesions that produce no obvious neurological deficits.

11.4.5 Endocarditis, myocarditis, pericarditis and other vascular infections

Candida infection is the most common form of fungal endocarditis. Three groups of individuals develop this condition: (i) patients with underlying native valve disease; (ii) patients with prosthetic heart valves; and (iii) intravenous drug abusers. The aortic and mitral valves are the most frequent sites of infection, but the tricuspid valve is often involved in drug abusers.

In surgical patients, endocarditis tends to occur within the first 2 months after the operation. The prognosis has been poor and more than 80% of patients given antifungal treatment alone have died. Earlier and improved surgical intervention has led to more patients surviving.

The symptoms and clinical signs are similar to those of bacterial endocarditis. The illness may be abrupt in onset or insidious. Fever, weight loss, fatigue and loss of appetite are common, but non-specific, symptoms. Heart murmurs can be detected in 50–90% of patients, and an enlarged spleen in 30–50%. More specific diagnostic signs include large vegetations, large vessel embolization and endophthalmitis.

Myocardial infection with abscess formation is a complication of endocarditis, but it may also occur as a result of haematogenous spread of organisms. It has been found in 50% of patients dying with disseminated candidosis. The diagnosis is difficult. Non-specific electrocardiogram (ECG) abnormalities are common.

Purulent pericarditis is an unusual complication of haematogenous dissemination of *Candida* infection. It can arise also from extension of a superficial myocardial abscess. The diagnostic signs are non-specific and include chest pain, pericardial friction rub and pericardial effusion.

Other vascular infections include septic thrombophlebitis of peripheral or central veins and prosthetic graft infections.

11.4.6 Renal candidosis

It is much more common for renal candidosis to result from the haematogenous spread of organisms than for it to occur as a result of ascending infection. At least 80% of patients with disseminated candidosis develop renal infection. For this reason, disseminated infection should be suspected in a febrile neutropenic patient with candiduria. Renal infection often results in abscess formation. Less commonly, it results in the formation of clumps of mycelium which can obstruct the pelvis or ureters leading to hydronephrosis or anuria.

The symptoms of renal candidosis include fever, rigors, lumbar pain and abdominal pain. Oliguria and anuria are common presenting signs in infants with this infection. There are no specific radiological signs, apart from fungus balls in the renal pelvis or ureters, which appear as radiolucent, irregular filling defects.

11.4.7 Lower urinary tract candidosis

Most of these infections are due to the local spread of organisms from an indwelling urethral catheter or from the genital or gastrointestinal tract. Infection is more common in women than men and tends to occur in diabetics or patients with abnormal or damaged urinary tracts. Many infections are related to an indwelling catheter. The clinical presentation is varied, but unlike those with bacterial infections, most patients with candiduria have no symptoms.

Although *C. albicans* is the most common organism, *C. glabrata* accounts for up to 30% of isolations from the urine. *C. glabrata* is often recovered from patients with urethral catheters and individuals with diabetes mellitus. It is often resistant to antifungal treatment (see Chapter 3).

11.4.8 Peritonitis

Candida peritonitis is an uncommon complication of peritoneal dialysis. It can also occur as a result of gastro-intestinal perforation or contamination from a leaking intestinal anastomosis. In surgical patients *Candida* perito-nitis is often associated with bacterial peritonitis. It may be insidious in onset.

The symptoms and signs are similar to those of bacterial peritonitis. The most common symptoms are abdominal pain and tenderness, with or without nausea or vomiting. Most patients have fever. *C. albicans* is the most common pathogen, but *C. tropicalis* and *C. parapsilosis* are some-times involved.

11.4.9 Intrauterine candidosis

Although symptomatic candidosis of the lower genital tract is one of the most common infections encountered in preg-nant women (see Chapter 5), fetal infection is unusual. Intrauterine candidosis is believed to result from ascending infection of the maternal genital tract. In most cases, fetal infection follows contamination of the amniotic fluid. Spontaneous abortion associated with fetal candidosis has been reported in women fitted with an intrauterine contra-ceptive device.

Intrauterine candidosis presents as multiple small yellow–white lesions scattered over the surface of the umbilical cord. In some cases the fungus affects the fetus and in live births such infections manifest as the characteristic lesions of congenital cutaneous candidosis (see Chapter 5). Umbi-lical cord lesions are often associated with other lesions which are less characteristic and take the form of diffuse, generalized chorioamnionitis.

11.4.10 Osteomyelitis, arthritis and myositis

Osteomyelitis is an uncommon form of candidosis. It usually occurs as a late complication of the haematogenous dissemination of organisms in neutropenic cancer patients and low birth-weight infants. It can also result from direct inoculation following surgical or accidental trauma. In adult

patients the lumbar spine is often involved. The commonest symptom is local pain, but fever is often absent. The infection gives rise to characteristic osteolytic lesions.

Arthritis is usually the result of haematogenous dissemination, but it can also result from the inadvertent inoculation of organisms into the joint during aspiration, or injection of corticosteroids, or during insertion of a prosthetic joint replacement. The symptoms include indolent joint pain and effusion. The large joints are most commonly involved.

Muscular tenderness is often associated with disseminated *C. tropicalis* infections in neutropenic patients.

11.4.11   Endophthalmitis

This sight-threatening ocular infection is increasing in incidence. It is an occasional complication of ocular trauma, but is more commonly seen following haematogenous dissemination of organisms. It is seldom encountered in neutropenic patients, but often occurs in intravenous drug abusers.

The symptoms include blurred vision, ocular pain and floaters. Fundoscopic examination will reveal the typical yellow–white retinal, chorioretinal, or vitreoretinal lesions with indistinct borders. The lesions may be unilateral or bilateral and can develop into a vitreous abscess. Extension into the anterior chamber may occur. In most cases, infection results in blindness unless treated.

11.4.12   Disseminated candidosis

This condition is not one disease: rather, it is a continuous spectrum of different patterns of infection which have different implications for treatment and prognosis. Three distinct patterns of infection can be distinguished: candidaemia, acute disseminated candidosis, and chronic disseminated candidosis. However, it is important to remember that many patients present with patterns of disease intermediate between these different forms.

CANDIDAEMIA

This is best defined as one or more positive blood cultures with no evidence of organ involvement. It occurs in both neutropenic and non-neutropenic patients. It is most commonly seen in individuals with indwelling vascular

catheters, although these are not necessarily the source of the organisms.

The most common presentation is fever (often greater than 38°C), but some patients develop rigors or even hypotension.

ACUTE DISSEMINATED CANDIDOSIS

This is a fulminant life-threatening infection which is encountered in both neutropenic and non-neutropenic patients. It often presents as a persistent fever that fails to respond to broad-spectrum antibacterial treatment. Other useful clinical signs include macronodular cutaneous lesions (seen in about 10% of neutropenic patients) and endophthalmitis (found in about 30% of non-neutropenic patients, but seldom seen in neutropenic individuals). Common complications include meningitis, brain abscess, renal abscess, myositis, myocarditis and endocarditis. Late complications include osteomyelitis and septic arthritis.

CHRONIC DISSEMINATED CANDIDOSIS

Chronic disseminated candidosis is an indolent illness which occurs in leukaemic patients who have regained an adequate neutrophil count after remission induction treatment. It has sometimes been called hepatosplenic candidosis, but lesions are found in other organs as well.

In most cases, the infection begins while the patient is neutropenic and presents as a persistent fever that fails to respond to antibacterial treatment. There are no discernible lesions in any organ, nor are there signs of infection in any particular organ. The neutrophil count then returns to normal, but the fever persists and is often associated with continuing weight loss.

The patient may complain of abdominal pain, and hepatic and/or splenic enlargement may be detected. Many patients have highly elevated blood levels of alkaline phosphatase, but other liver function abnormalities may be mild or absent. The diagnosis should be suspected if CT scans reveal numerous, small radiolucent lesions in the liver or spleen.

Microscopic examination of stained sections of biopsied tissue will often confirm the diagnosis, but the organism is isolated from no more than 30% of specimens. Blood

cultures are negative. *C. albicans* is the principal aetiological agent, but *C. tropicalis* has sometimes been implicated.

11.5 Candidosis in special hosts

11.5.1 Low birth-weight infants

Unifocal and multifocal forms of deep-seated candidosis can occur in low birth-weight infants requiring prolonged neonatal intensive care. Meningitis occurs more frequently than in older patients and is sometimes associated with arthritis and osteomyelitis. Although uncommon, isolated renal infection can also occur and result in ureteric obstruction and renal failure. Prolonged vascular catheterization, tracheal intubation, parenteral nutrition and broad-spectrum antibacterial treatment are among the important risk factors for disseminated candidosis in low birth-weight infants.

11.5.2 Drug abusers

Addicts who inject heroin solutions contaminated with *C. albicans* often develop an unusual form of disseminated candidosis. This consists of a purulent follicular and nodular cutaneous infection associated with ocular and osteoarticular lesions. The symptoms include sudden onset of fever, rigors, headache and myalgia several hours after the injection of heroin. The fever lasts between 24 and 72 h and cutaneous lesions then appear in more than 90% of patients. Endophthalmitis develops in 40–60% of patients, occurring 1–2 weeks after the onset of fever. Osteoarticular lesions develop in 20–30% of patients, appearing 2 weeks to several months after the cutaneous lesions. Costochondral involvement is a frequent and characteristic finding.

11.5.3 Patients with AIDS

Oral infection with *C. albicans* (see Chapter 5) often spreads to the oesophagus in human immunodeficiency virus (HIV)-positive individuals. Oesophagitis can also occur without oral involvement, but this is unusual. Oesophageal candidosis is an important AIDS-defining diagnosis: it has been the AIDS-defining illness in 10–15% of North American patients with HIV infection. Other localized forms of deep candidosis, such as meningitis and endophthalmitis, have been reported, but widespread disseminated infection is

uncommon. In the few patients with AIDS who have developed this condition, prolonged vascular catheterization has been an important predisposing factor.

One consequence of the widespread use of fluconazole in patients with AIDS with oesophageal candidosis has been a growing number of reports describing the development of resistance to this agent among the *C. albicans* strains recovered from these patients. In most cases the individuals concerned had received repeated courses of antifungal treatment.

11.6 Essential investigations and their interpretation

Establishing the diagnosis of deep-seated candidosis is difficult because the clinical presentation is non-specific and because the results of microbiological and serological tests are difficult to interpret. In cases of suspected deep-seated candidosis, cultures should be made from as many sources as possible and efforts should also be made to obtain material for histopathological examination.

11.6.1 Microscopy

The detection of typical blastospore or filamentous forms of *Candida* species in stained tissue sections is diagnostic of deep-seated candidosis.

11.6.2 Culture

Many members of the genus *Candida* are normal commensal inhabitants of the mouth and gastrointestinal tract and their isolation from sputum or faecal specimens cannot be considered diagnostic of infection. Isolation from blood or other fluids, or from other closed sites, or from macronodular cutaneous lesions provides more reliable evidence of deep-seated infection. It is important that specimens are processed as soon as possible after collection to avoid problems of interpretation because of multiplication of organisms. It is recommended that all isolates from blood or other significant sites are speciated before commencing treatment.

Blood culture should be performed in all cases of suspected deep-seated candidosis. However, it is not unusual for numerous attempts to be required before the organism is recovered. Blood should be drawn both through intravenous catheters and from peripheral veins. Lysis-centrifugation is a more sensitive technique than culture in vented

biphasic media or broth. Blood cultures are positive in no more than 50% of neutropenic patients with disseminated candidosis or 80% of patients with endocarditis.

Isolation of *Candida* from urine is often indicative of serious infection, provided the patient does not have an indwelling urethral catheter. In non-catheterized patients, care must be taken to ensure that vaginal or perineal infection does not lead to contamination of urine specimens. In infants, suprapubic aspiration is the best method of urine collection. Isolation of *C. tropicalis* from urine is more often indicative of disseminated candidosis than isolation of *C. albicans*. It has been suggested that counts of > 1 × 10^4 cfu/ml in a non-catheterized patient should be regarded as significant, but this has never been validated. High counts in a patient with an indwelling catheter are seldom significant.

Isolation of *Candida* from the CSF provides reliable evidence for the diagnosis of meningitis, but often requires repeated culture of large amounts of fluid. All specimens obtained from ventricular shunts or reservoirs should be cultured for *Candida* species.

Particular care must be taken in interpreting the results of sputum culture as this material is often contaminated with organisms from the mouth. Isolation of *Candida* from bronchoalveolar lavage in a patient with pulmonary infiltrates is not sufficient to establish a diagnosis of candidosis. Lung biopsies provide more reliable evidence of infection.

11.6.3 Serological tests

Serological tests should be attempted in all cases of suspected deep-seated candidosis, although the results must be interpreted with care. A single positive precipitin test result is not diagnostic of infection because the mannan and somatic antigens used are unable to distinguish antibodies formed during deep infection from those produced during mucosal colonization or infection. Nor does a negative precipitin test result preclude the diagnosis of deep candidosis in an immunocompromised patient, because such individuals are often incapable of mounting a detectable antibody response.

Tests for the detection of *Candida* antibodies are most useful when sequential serum specimens are tested at intervals over a period of time. High or rising antibody titres should be regarded as suspicious.

Tests for the detection of antibodies are least helpful in immunocompromised patients. In such cases, methods for the detection of *Candida* antigen may be more useful. However, a negative antigen test result does not preclude the diagnosis of candidosis, particularly if only a single specimen has been tested and the patient has clinical signs or other findings consistent with the infection.

Numerous reports have described attempts to detect circulating *Candida* mannan, a heat-stable cell wall component, in patients with deep-seated candidosis. However, as mannan is rapidly cleared from the circulation and the serum concentration is low, frequent sampling is essential if the antigen is to be detected. Latex particle agglutination tests for detection of *Candida* mannan are available.

The development of immunoblotting methods has permitted the identification of a number of immunodominant antigens of *Candida albicans*. Among these are a 48-kDa antigen, that has been identified as an enolase, and a 47-kDa antigen which is a product of a 90-kDa heat shock protein. Both antigens have been detected in serum specimens from neutropenic cancer patients with deep-seated candidosis. Tests for these antigens are available from some specialist laboratories.

11.7 Management

11.7.1 Oesophagitis

Oesophageal candidosis can be treated with oral ketoconazole (200–400 mg/day for 1–2 weeks) or fluconazole (100–200 mg/day for 1–2 weeks). Oral itraconazole (200–400 mg/day for 2 weeks) is also effective, but this drug is less reliably absorbed than fluconazole. Administration of the oral solution formulation of itraconazole has proved successful in patients who failed to respond to the capsule formulation. Patients who remain symptomatic after 2 weeks require further investigation for drug resistance, drug interactions and other causes of oesophagitis.

Management of oesophagitis in patients with AIDS from whom fluconazole-resistant strains of *C. albicans* have been isolated is difficult. Higher doses of fluconazole (400–800 mg/day) should be tried, but the benefit is often transient. Itraconazole solution (400 mg/day) can be prescribed, as this has sometimes proved successful in patients who had failed to respond to fluconazole. However, it is not unreasonable to expect these patients to need higher than usual doses of itraconazole.

As a last resort, patients with azole-resistant oesophagitis can be managed with parenteral amphotericin B (0.5–0.7 mg/kg per day for 1 week). However, relapse is common and intermittent maintenance treatment (1 mg/kg twice or three times per week) may be required.

11.7.2   **Meningitis**

Meningitis in neurosurgical patients and low birth-weight infants is best treated with amphotericin B (1.0 mg/kg per day) and flucytosine (100–150 mg/kg per day) (provided the infecting organism is susceptible). The half-life of flucytosine is prolonged in small infants and the drug should be administered at 12- or 24-h intervals. Infected shunts should be removed or replaced. Fluconazole (200–400 mg/day, or 5 mg/kg in infants) is a useful alternative treatment.

11.7.3   **Endocarditis and vascular infection**

The management of fungal endocarditis is difficult. Treatment with amphotericin B (1.0 mg/kg per day) and flucytosine (100–150 mg/kg per day) (provided the organism is susceptible) should be commenced as soon as the diagnosis is made. Infected valves should be replaced 1–2 weeks after treatment has started, but earlier surgical intervention is indicated if there are large vegetations, signs of heart failure, or dysfunction of a prosthesis. The optimum length of treatment remains uncertain, but 2–3 months has been recommended to reduce the likelihood of relapse.

Treatment with a lipid-based formulation of amphotericin B should be considered in patients who fail to respond to the conventional formulation, or who develop side-effects that necessitate discontinuation of the drug, or in whom conventional amphotericin B is contraindicated because of renal impairment. There is insufficient experience with fluconazole to recommend it as a first-line treatment.

Unlike endocarditis, septic central vein thrombosis is often curable with antifungal treatment alone. The catheter should be removed and amphotericin B given for 1–2 months; flucytosine can be added during the initial phase of treatment. Anticoagulation is desirable, but not essential for a successful outcome. Septic thrombophlebitis at a peripheral site requires resection of the vein in addition to amphotericin B treatment.

11.7.4 Renal candidosis

There are three basic approaches to the management of renal candidosis: (i) local irrigation of the renal pelvis with antifungal drugs; (ii) oral or parenteral treatment with antifungals; and (iii) surgical removal of obstructions or resection. In practice, a combined approach is often required.

Amphotericin B (1.0 mg/kg per day), with or without flucytosine (100–150 mg/kg per day), remains the treatment of choice for renal candidosis. Fluconazole is excreted unchanged and in high concentrations in the urine. Its use is still under evaluation, but it is a useful alternative to amphotericin B, provided the infecting organism is susceptible. It should not be used to treat *C. glabrata* or *C. krusei* infections. The recommended dose of fluconazole is 200–400 mg/day, but this may need to be modified in patients with impaired renal function (see Chapter 3).

11.7.5 Lower urinary tract candidosis

Local instillation of an antifungal drug is reasonable in individuals with persistent candiduria related to an indwelling urethral catheter, provided there are no signs of pyelonephritis, or of renal or ureteric obstruction. These patients often respond following catheter change and intermittent instillation (200–300 ml of a 50 mg/l solution in sterile water at 6–8-h intervals) or continuous irrigation with amphotericin B (50 mg/l in sterile water) for 5–7 days. Oral treatment with fluconazole (100–200 mg/day) for 2–4 weeks is the simplest and best option for cystitis in patients without indwelling catheters. However, it should not be used to treat *C. glabrata* or *C. krusei* infections.

11.7.6 Peritonitis

Patients receiving peritoneal dialysis should have their catheter removed as soon as possible and should be started on parenteral amphotericin B treatment (1.0 mg/kg per day for at least 2 weeks), with or without flucytosine (100–150 mg/kg per day), and haemodialysis (if required). If the dialysate is grossly turbid, peritoneal lavage (until the returning fluid is clear) should be performed before the catheter is removed. It can be replaced once antifungal treatment has been discontinued.

If the infecting organism is susceptible to fluconazole, this drug can be used instead of amphotericin B. The recommended dosage is 200–400 mg/day for 2–4 weeks.

Patients who are diagnosed as having *Candida* peritonitis within 2 weeks of starting dialysis can sometimes be managed without catheter removal, provided their symptoms and clinical signs are mild. Patients who cannot have their catheter removed should be treated with amphotericin B or fluconazole, depending on the organism. Intraperitoneal administration of amphotericin B is painful, but may need to be considered. The peritoneal catheter should be removed as soon as the patient can be managed with haemodialysis.

Amphotericin B (1.0 mg/kg per day), with or without flucytosine (100–150 mg/kg per day), remains the drug of choice for surgical patients with *Candida* peritonitis. Fluconazole (200–400 mg/day) is a useful alternative treatment. Peritonitis arising from perforation first requires surgical repair.

11.7.7 Osteomyelitis and arthritis

Amphotericin B (1.0 mg/kg per day), with or without flucytosine (100–150 mg/kg per day) remains the treatment of choice for osteomyelitis. Debridement of necrotic bone (with bone grafting at the same procedure) is recommended if extensive vertebral destruction is present. Fluconazole (200–400 mg/day) is a useful alternative treatment.

In patients with infected non-prosthetic joints, parenteral amphotericin B (1.0 mg/kg per day) is the most appropriate treatment. If there is no improvement within a week, flucytosine (100–150 mg/kg per day) can be added (provided the organism is susceptible). Intra-articular injection of amphotericin B is seldom required. In patients with prosthetic joints, treatment involves replacement of the joint together with removal of all foreign material and necrotic bone tissue. This is often difficult and long-term maintenance treatment with an azole may be an alternative, particularly in older patients.

11.7.8 Endophthalmitis

This is best treated with amphotericin B (1.0 mg/kg per day) and flucytosine (100–150 mg/kg per day) (provided the organism is susceptible). Fluconazole (400 mg/day) reaches high concentrations in the vitreous humour, but until there is more experience with this agent, it is difficult to recommend it as first-line treatment.

Large progressive lesions usually require surgical intervention and intravitreal dosing with amphotericin B. The drug is toxic, but two or three intravitreal doses (of 5 μg each) can be tolerated. Subconjunctival treatment with amphotericin B is not required.

11.7.9 Acute disseminated candidosis and candidaemia

All patients with candidaemia require treatment, regardless of whether or not this is associated with an intravascular catheter, and whether or not the patient is neutropenic. Treatment should be started at once, without waiting for confirmation from further cultures.

Non-neutropenic patients can be treated with amphotericin B (1.0 mg/kg per day of the conventional formulation) or fluconazole (400 mg/day), depending in part on the infecting organism. In patients with a life-threatening infection, the full dose of amphotericin B (50 mg) can be given from the outset (see Chapter 3). These patients should also receive flucytosine (100–150 mg/kg per day), provided the organism is susceptible.

Treatment with a lipid-based formulation of amphotericin B should be considered in patients who fail to respond to the conventional parenteral formulation, or who develop side-effects, or in whom conventional amphotericin B is contraindicated because of renal impairment.

If the response to amphotericin B is rapid or if the patient was less seriously ill at the outset, it is reasonable to change to fluconazole (400 mg/day) after 1–2 weeks.

It is still unclear whether fluconazole is as effective as amphotericin B in treating neutropenic patients, or whether it is safe to start treatment with amphotericin B and then change to fluconazole. It is reasonable to use fluconazole (400 mg/day) in neutropenic patients who have no signs of disseminated infection, provided the infecting organism is susceptible, and provided the patient has not been receiving prophylactic treatment with an azole. Amphotericin B (1.0 mg/kg per day), with or without flucytosine (100–150 mg/kg per day) should be used in all other situations.

Intravascular catheters must be changed or removed in both neutropenic and non-neutropenic patients, whenever this is feasible. If it is not possible to replace long-term tunnelled catheters, amphotericin B and not fluconazole should be used.

The regimen of choice for neonatal candidosis is the combination of amphotericin B (1.0 mg/kg per day) and flucytosine (100–150 mg/kg per day) (provided the infecting organism is susceptible). The latter drug is useful because of the high incidence of meningitis in this age group. The half-life of flucytosine is prolonged in small infants and the drug should be administered at 12- or 24-h intervals. Fluconazole (5 mg/kg) is a useful alternative treatment.

The shortcomings of current methods of diagnosis often require clinicians to proceed to amphotericin B treatment without waiting for formal proof that a neutropenic patient with persistent fever (> 72–96 h duration), resistant to antibacterial drugs, has a fungal infection. Empirical treatment should be initiated with the usual test dose (1 mg) of amphotericin B. If possible, the full therapeutic dosage level (1.0 mg/kg per day of the conventional formulation) should be reached within the first 24 h of treatment. There is no need for gradual escalation of dosage, nor is there evidence to support the clinical prejudice that a lower dose can be used in suspected candidosis (see Chapter 3). Should the conventional formulation be contraindicated, one of the lipid-based formulations should be used instead.

Prophylactic treatment with fluconazole (100–200 mg/day) has been shown to reduce the incidence of colonization and infection with all *Candida* species, apart from *C. glabrata* and *C. krusei*, in neutropenic cancer patients, in BMT recipients and in liver transplant patients. Itraconazole (400 mg/day) is also effective (see Chapter 3 for a discussion of the role of prophylactic treatment). It is unclear at present whether other groups of high-risk patients should be offered prophylaxis.

11.7.10   Chronic disseminated candidosis

The usual treatment for chronic disseminated candidosis (hepatosplenic candidosis) in cancer patients has been amphotericin B (1.0 mg/kg per day), but the infection often persists despite the administration of this drug for periods of 6 months to total doses of as high as 5 g. Liposomal amphotericin B (AmBisome) has been more promising. Administration of the drug in this form at dosages of 3–5 mg/kg per day has eradicated hepatosplenic infection and permitted the resumption of antineoplastic treatment in some leukaemic patients. Administration of oral fluconazole, at dosages of 400 mg/day or higher, has also proved successful in a small number of patients with hepatosplenic candidosis.

12   Cryptococcosis

12.1   Definition

The term cryptococcosis is used to refer to infections due to the encapsulated yeast *Cryptococcus neoformans*. This ubiquitous organism can cause disease in normal individuals, but a high proportion of human infections occur in immunocompromised patients. Infection follows inhalation, but meningitis is the most common clinical presentation and widespread disseminated infection can also occur.

12.2   Geographical distribution

The condition is worldwide in distribution.

12.3   The causal organism and its habitat

Two varieties of *C. neoformans* are recognized: var. *neoformans* and var. *gattii*. Each of these can be divided into two serological groups, A and D, and B and C. There have been reports of human infections due to *C. albidus* and *C. laurentii*, but the significance of these isolations remains doubtful.

The two varieties of *C. neoformans* differ in their natural habitat and geographical distribution. *C. neoformans* var. *neoformans* has a global distribution, but *C. neoformans* var. *gattii* is restricted to tropical and subtropical regions. Although *C. neoformans* var. *neoformans* has often been isolated from the environment (from old, dried accumulations of pigeon droppings and soil contaminated with bird droppings), it was not until 1990 that the natural habitat of *C. neoformans* var. *gattii* was identified as the red gum tree, *Eucalyptus camaldulensis*, whose global distribution coincides with that of var. *gattii* infection in humans. It is notable that, despite the occurrence of the acquired immune deficiency syndrome (AIDS) in regions (such as central Africa) that are endemic for *C. neoformans* var. *gattii*, this variety is a rare cause of cryptococcosis in patients with AIDS.

Inhalation of *C. neoformans* is believed to be the usual mode of infection in humans. The infectious particles could be small desiccated acapsular cells disseminated in the air from accumulations of dried bird droppings, or basidiospores of the perfect form of the fungus, *Filobasidiella neoformans*.

Until the 1980s, cryptococcosis was an uncommon and sporadic infection which tended to occur in individuals with T-cell mediated immunological defects, such as patients with cancer, organ transplant recipients and individuals receiving corticosteroid treatment. Now it has become a major cause of illness and death among patients with AIDS, and is one of the most common causes of meningitis in hospitals where these patients are treated.

12.4   Clinical manifestations

Most cases of cryptococcosis are not diagnosed until signs of meningitis have appeared. However, it is well established that the lungs are the usual initial site of involvement. In most patients, infection of the lungs occurs and resolves weeks to months before disseminated infection is detected.

12.4.1   Pulmonary cryptococcosis

Up to 30% of normal individuals develop no symptoms following inhalation of *C. neoformans* and their infection remains unrecognized until it has spread to other organs. However, the remainder present with symptoms, such as cough, chest pain, sputum production, weight loss and fever. The most frequent radiological findings are well-defined, non-calcified, single or multiple nodular lesions. Less common findings include indistinct to mass-like infiltrates, hilar and mediastinal lymph node enlargement, pleural effusions and cavitation.

In immunocompromised individuals, cryptococcosis of the lungs follows a much more rapid course and patients often present with disseminated infection. Unlike normal individuals, most immunocompromised patients present with symptoms. The most common are fever, malaise, chest pain, weight loss, dyspnoea, night sweats and cough. Chest radiographs will reveal diffuse interstitial or alveolar infiltrates. Nodular lesions, pleural effusions and cavitation are sometimes found.

Although pulmonary infection is a much less common initial presentation than meningitis in patients with AIDS with cryptococcosis, these individuals often develop more persistent infection than other patients. The clinical manifestations differ somewhat from those found in other groups of immunocompromised patients. Almost all patients with AIDS present with symptoms, including fever, cough, dyspnoea, weight loss and headache. Occasional patients present with pleuritic chest pain and haemoptysis. Chest radiographs will often reveal focal or diffuse interstitial infiltrates and hilar lymph node enlargement. Unlike other patients, nodular and alveolar infiltrates are rare. Large mass lesions and pleural effusions are also unusual.

Most patients with AIDS in whom cryptococcosis of the lungs is diagnosed have disseminated infection: 60–70% have concurrent meningeal involvement. The organism can be isolated from sputum, bronchoalveolar lavage (BAL) fluid and tissue biopsies, as well as blood and other specimens. Antigen can often be detected in BAL fluid as well as serum, urine and cerebrospinal fluid (CSF) specimens.

12.4.2 Meningitis

Infection of the brain and meninges is the most common clinical form of cryptococcosis and the most frequent cause of death. It follows dissemination of the organism from the lungs.

In patients without AIDS the symptoms and signs are often indolent in onset. Headache is the most common presenting symptom: the pain is dull, bilateral and diffuse. Fever is often minimal or absent until late in the course of the infection. Mental changes, such as drowsiness and confusion, also occur. Hydrocephalus is a serious complication, but focal neurological lesions are uncommon. These lesions are insidious in onset and present with focal signs. Computed tomographic (CT) scans will reveal single or multiple, enhancing or non-enhancing nodular lesions.

About 90% of patients have abnormal CSF findings including increased pressure, raised protein concentration, lowered glucose concentration and a lymphocytic pleocytosis.

In patients with AIDS, meningeal infection with *C. neoformans* is often insidious in onset. Headache and fever are common, but overt meningeal symptoms and signs are unusual: fewer than 20% of patients are somnolent, confused or obtunded. Focal neurological signs are uncommon on initial presentation, occurring in about 10% of patients. If focal neurological lesions are detected on CT or magnetic resonance imaging (MRI) scans, a second disease (such as another infection) should be considered.

Patients with AIDS with cryptococcal meningitis often develop symptoms of increased intracranial pressure, such as increasing headache, lowered consciousness and visual loss, soon after starting antifungal treatment. This can result in a rapid deterioration in their condition and death. The underlying mechanism is unclear, but accumulation of dead organisms in the subarachnoid space following treatment might reduce CSF outflow and lead to elevation in intracranial pressure. Serial measurements of opening pressure at the time of lumbar puncture and treatment of raised CSF pressure are critical factors in successful management. In obtunded or somnolent patients a repeat lumbar puncture should be done within 1 week of starting treatment to check the CSF pressure.

12.4.3 Cutaneous cryptococcosis

Haematogenous spread of *C. neoformans* gives rise to cutaneous lesions in 10–15% of patients with disseminated cryptococcosis. In some cases these lesions are the earliest clinical sign of infection. They are often located on the head, but may occur on the trunk or limbs. The lesions may present as single or multiple nodules, ulcers or abscesses.

Cutaneous lesions are common in patients with AIDS with cryptococcosis. Multiple small maculopapular lesions, some of which show central necrotic umbilication resembling molluscum contagiosum, are frequently reported. Microscopic examination and culture of biopsied material from a suspicious lesion should permit the diagnosis to be established.

12.4.4 Osteomyelitis

Osteomyelitis occurs in 5–10% of patients with disseminated cryptococcosis. Most patients present with a single isolated lesion, the most common site of involvement being the spine. Patients complain of local pain and soft-tissue tenderness at the affected site. Radiographs will reveal well-defined osteolytic lesions without marginal sclerosis or periosteal change. CT scans can be used to define the extent of bone involvement. Microscopic examination and culture of aspirated or biopsied material from a suspicious lesion should permit the diagnosis to be established.

12.4.5

Other forms of cryptococcosis

Ocular infection with *C. neoformans* is not uncommon, occurring in up to 40% of patients with meningitis. In some cases endophthalmitis is present before the diagnosis of meningitis is made. Prompt diagnosis and rapid treatment are essential to prevent visual loss. Catastrophic visual loss has also been reported in patients with AIDS without endophthalmitis. In some cases visual loss has occurred over a period as short as 12 h. Others have presented with slower visual loss related to raised intracranial pressure following central nervous system (CNS) infection.

Asymptomatic infection of the prostate is common in patients with AIDS with cryptococcosis. Moreover, cultures of urine and prostatic secretions often remain positive following apparently successful antifungal treatment of meningitis and other disseminated forms of cryptococcosis. It is clear that the prostate is an important reservoir for relapse of infection.

Other unusual sites of infection include the adrenal gland, heart, liver and spleen.

12.5

Cryptococcosis in special hosts

12.5.1

Patients with AIDS

Cryptococcosis is the most important life-threatening fungal complication in patients with AIDS. The incidence of this infection differs from one continent to another, ranging from around 5–10% in European, North American and Australian patients with AIDS, to 15–30% in Africans. In the USA the infection appears to be more frequent among African-American patients with AIDS than among those from other racial groups.

The clinical manifestations of cryptococcosis in patients with AIDS are similar to those in other groups of immunocompromised individuals. However, infected sites often contain a much higher burden of organisms. More than 80% of patients with AIDS have meningitis or meningoencephalitis at the time of diagnosis, but the disease is often more widespread. Because the clinical presentation can be so non-specific it is important to consider the diagnosis in all patients with AIDS who present with a fever and to reevaluate them at regular intervals for cryptococcal infection, even if the initial investigations are negative.

Patients with AIDS with cryptococcosis can seldom be cured and persistent or recurrent infection is usual. Ten to twenty-five per cent of these individuals will die during their initial treatment and 30–60% within 12 months.

12.6 Essential investigations and their interpretation

Establishing the diagnosis of cryptococcosis is less difficult than diagnosis of other fungal infections.

12.6.1 Microscopy

Encapsulated *C. neoformans* cells can often be detected in specimens of CSF or other host fluids or secretions mounted in Indian ink or nigrosin. However, lymphocytes in particular can be confused with the organism. In patients with AIDS, *C. neoformans* cells are usually plentiful in the CSF, although the capsules are often small making recognition difficult. Persistently positive CSF findings in patients undergoing treatment should be considered evidence of failure or relapse only if they are confirmed by a deterioration in the patient's clinical condition or by positive cultures.

12.6.2 Culture

The likelihood of isolating *C. neoformans* from CSF is increased if multiple specimens are taken and the centrifuged sediment of large amounts (4–8 ml) of fluid are plated out. The organism grows best at 30–35°C and it is advisable to prolong incubation of plates in suspected cases for up to 2 weeks.

C. neoformans can also be recovered from blood, sputum, urine, prostatic fluid and other specimens. Positive blood cultures have been obtained in 35–70% of patients with AIDS with cryptococcosis. Lysis-centrifugation has been the most sensitive method. Because of the greater load of organisms, microscopic examination and culture of other specimens is more often positive in untreated patients with AIDS than in other individuals.

12.6.3 Serological tests

Antibodies to *C. neoformans* can often be detected in

patients with early or localized infection, but are seldom found in patients with untreated meningeal or disseminated infection in whom tests for antigen are much more helpful.

Testing for *C. neoformans* capsular antigen is one of the most reliable methods for the diagnosis of cryptococcosis. Several latex particle agglutination (LPA) and enzyme-linked immunoadsorbent assay (ELISA) tests have been marketed for the detection of antigen in serum, CSF, urine and BAL fluid specimens. These tests are specific, provided that rheumatoid and other interfering factors are removed. False-negative results can occur if the organism load is low or if the organisms are not well encapsulated. It is also important to remember that different manufacturers' products can give different titres with the same clinical specimen.

Antigen tests should be performed on all CSF specimens taken at the time of diagnosis as well as on subsequent CSF specimens as one means of evaluating the response to treatment. Serum antigen levels are also useful in monitoring the response to treatment, provided they are used in conjunction with clinical evaluation of the patient. Their main advantage over CSF antigen levels is that blood can more easily and frequently be obtained. Changes in titre of less than fourfold are not considered significant.

A negative serum antigen test result does not exclude the diagnosis of cryptococcosis, particularly if only a single specimen has been tested and the patient has symptoms consistent with the infection. Repeated negative test results for serum antigen in patients with AIDS without neurological symptoms or signs makes the diagnosis improbable, but should not preclude the clinician who still suspects cryptococcal meningitis from performing a lumbar puncture.

The antigen test is positive in over 90% of patients with untreated meningeal infection. Much higher LPA titres in both serum (greater than 1:1000 000) and CSF (greater than 1:64 000) have been detected in patients with AIDS. Levels of antigen in the CSF often decline with treatment, but the test may remain positive for several weeks. This is more common in patients whose initial load of organisms is high. Positive CSF antigen test results may be obtained despite failure to recover *C. neoformans* from the CSF. This may represent the persistent release of antigen from dead cells or slow elimination of capsular antigen from the CSF, rather than ongoing infection.

In patients without AIDS high levels of serum and CSF antigen prior to treatment are often predictive of death during treatment. In patients with AIDS abnormal mental status prior to treatment is the most important factor, but a high CSF antigen titre (greater than 1 : 1000) is also a sign of a poor prognosis.

In patients without AIDS high antigen levels at the end of treatment are often predictive of later relapse. In contrast, in patients with AIDS measurement of antigen levels at the end of initial acute treatment has not been predictive of relapse. However, an unchanging or rising CSF antigen titre is often associated with failure of acute treatment and with relapse during maintenance treatment.

12.7 Management

All patients with cryptococcosis, apart from a few non-compromised individuals with infection of the lungs, require treatment.

12.7.1 Meningitis and disseminated infection

Patients presenting with meningitis should be investigated for signs of disseminated cryptococcosis. In addition to physical examination, CSF, blood, urine and prostatic fluid should be cultured, and CSF and blood should be tested for antigen. These investigations should be repeated at intervals until the patient recovers.

NON-AIDS PATIENTS

The standard treatment for patients with meningeal or disseminated infection is the combination of amphotericin B (0.3–0.5 mg/kg per day) and flucytosine (100–150 mg/kg per day). In patients with a life-threatening infection, the full dose of amphotericin B (50 mg) can be given from the outset (see Chapter 3). In immunocompromised patients, the combination regimen should be given for at least 6 weeks. In non-compromised individuals, it may be effective when given for 4 weeks. Flucytosine concentrations should be monitored at regular intervals.

If there is significant deterioration in the patient's condition after treatment is initiated, or if there is no clinical improvement after 3 weeks of treatment, the dose of amphotericin B should be increased to 0.6–1.0 mg/kg per day. If the patient is receiving corticosteroids, the steroid dosage should be reduced. Patients with elevated CSF pressure require pressure-reducing measures, such as lumbar punctures, a lumbar drain or a ventricular shunt.

If amphotericin B is given on its own, it should be administered in a higher dose (0.8–1.0 mg/kg per day) than that used in the combination regimen. At least 10 weeks of treatment is often required.

Itraconazole and fluconazole are less toxic than amphotericin B, but the role of these drugs in the treatment of cryptococcosis in patients without AIDS is unclear at present. The suggested dose of both azoles is 400 mg/day and this should be continued for at least 6–8 weeks.

The decision to discontinue treatment should be based on clinical examination and the results of mycological and antigen tests. Lumbar punctures should be performed at 1-week intervals for the first 6 weeks of treatment. The return of CSF white cell counts, and protein and glucose levels to normal is helpful, but less reliable.

In addition to physical examination, blood and CSF specimens should be cultured and tested for antigen 1, 2, 3 and 6 months after treatment has ceased and thereafter at 12-month intervals.

PATIENTS WITH AIDS
Patients with AIDS with alterations in mental status should be treated with the combination of amphotericin B (at least 0.7 mg/kg per day of the conventional formulation) and flucytosine (100 mg/kg per day) for at least 2 weeks. Thereafter, if the patient has improved, high-dose fluconazole (400 mg/day) should be given for a further 8–10 weeks.

Patients who have not responded after 2 weeks should continue on amphotericin B treatment (at a higher dose) as should those who presented while taking oral azole treatment. It is unusual for more than 6 weeks of amphotericin B treatment to be required, provided follow-on azole treatment is given.

Administration of one of the lipid-based forms of amphotericin B should be considered in patients who develop side-effects that necessitate discontinuation of the conventional formulation, or in whom conventional amphotericin B is contraindicated because of renal impairment. There are different dosage recommendations for the various lipid-based preparations (see Chapter 3). These formulations have given comparable response rates to the conventional form in small numbers of patients.

Patients with elevated CSF pressure require pressure-reducing measures. These include frequent lumbar punctures (removing 25–30 ml of CSF on each occasion), oral acetazolamide treatment, or insertion of a lumbar drain or ventricular shunt. Corticosteroid treatment is not now recommended.

Patients with AIDS with normal mental status can sometimes be treated with oral fluconazole (400 mg/day) or itraconazole (400 mg/day) from the outset. However, the response rates at the end of treatment with these agents are lower than with parenteral amphotericin B treatment. It is recommended that all patients be given amphotericin B for 2 weeks (with flucytosine) before using itraconazole or fluconazole.

In recent trials combination treatment with fluconazole (400 mg/day) and flucytosine (150 mg/kg per day) has given encouraging results in small numbers of patients. More extensive evaluations of this combination are now in progress.

More than 50% of patients with AIDS with cryptococcosis relapse within 12 months of completing their initial treatment for acute disease. This potential for relapse necessitates long-term maintenance treatment. The drug of choice is fluconazole (200 mg/day) as this has proven superior to itraconazole (200 mg/day). The dose of fluconazole may need to be increased in patients receiving rifampicin or other enzyme-inducing drugs (see Chapter 3). To date there have been few reports of resistant strains of *C. neoformans* developing during long-term fluconazole treatment.

Patients who have undergone successful treatment often relapse because of persistence of *C. neoformans* in the prostate. This site is asymptomatic, but it often appears to account for relapses of infection in patients receiving maintenance treatment with less than 200 mg/day fluconazole and indicates the need for higher dosing regimens.

12.7.2 Pulmonary cryptococcosis

All patients with proven or suspected infection should be

investigated for signs of disseminated cryptococcosis. In addition to full physical examination (with particular attention to CNS function, hepatic or splenic enlargements and cutaneous rashes), CSF, blood, urine and prostatic fluid should be cultured, and CSF and blood should be tested for antigen. These investigations should be repeated at intervals until the patient recovers.

Immunocompromised patients should be treated to prevent progression or dissemination of infection. Treatment with amphotericin B or an azole is also required should symptoms persist for more than 3 weeks.

12.7.3 Cutaneous cryptococcosis

All patients with cutaneous cryptococcosis should be investigated for signs of disseminated infection. Lumbar puncture should be performed and radiographs of the underlying bone obtained. Blood and CSF should be tested for antigen. However, if the cutaneous lesion is the only manifestation of infection, the antigen test may well be negative.

If there is only one cutaneous lesion, surgical removal may be sufficient. However, it is advisable to give antifungal treatment with amphotericin B or an azole.

13 Mucormycosis

13.1 Definition

The term mucormycosis (zygomycosis) is used to refer to infections due to moulds belonging to the order Mucorales. These organisms can cause rhinocerebral, pulmonary, gastrointestinal, cutaneous or disseminated infection in predisposed individuals, the different clinical forms often being associated with particular underlying disorders.

13.2 Geographical distribution

These infections are worldwide in distribution.

13.3 The causal organisms and their habitat

Many different organisms have been implicated, but the most common cause of human infection is *Rhizopus arrhizus*. Other less frequent aetiological agents include *Absidia corymbifera*, *Apophysomyces elegans*, *Cunninghamella bertholletiae*, *Rhizomucor pusillus* and *Saksenaea vasiformis*. These moulds are ubiquitous, being found in the soil, in food and on decomposing organic matter. Their spores can often be found in the outside air.

Most human infections follow inhalation of spores that have been released into the air and the lungs and nasal sinuses are the most common initial sites of infection. Less frequently, infection follows ingestion or traumatic inoculation of organisms into the skin.

Nosocomial outbreaks of mucormycosis are not as common as hospital-related *Aspergillus* infections, but have been reported in neutropenic cancer patients. Hospital-acquired cutaneous infections with *R. rhizopodiformis* and *R. microsporus* have been traced to contaminated surgical dressings and splints.

The major risk factors predisposing individuals to mucormycosis include uncontrolled diabetes mellitus, other forms of metabolic acidosis, burns, and neutropenia. Treatment is seldom of benefit unless these underlying disorders can be corrected.

13.4 Clinical manifestations

Mucormycosis is an opportunistic infection and is seldom seen in normal persons. Various forms are recognized, each of which is associated with particular underlying disorders. Like the aetiological agents of aspergillosis, the causal organisms of mucormycosis have a predilection for vascular invasion causing thrombosis, infarction and necrosis of tissue. The clinical hallmark of mucormycosis is the rapid onset of necrosis and fever. In most cases, progress is rapid and death follows unless aggressive treatment is initiated.

13.4.1 Rhinocerebral mucormycosis

The terms rhinocerebral and craniofacial mucormycosis are used to describe an infection that begins in the paranasal sinuses and then spreads to involve the orbit, face, palate and/or brain. This condition is most commonly seen in acidotic individuals, particularly those with uncontrolled diabetes mellitus, but it also occurs in neutropenic cancer patients and solid organ transplant recipients. It is the most common clinical form of mucormycosis and often fatal within a week of onset if left untreated.

The initial symptoms include unilateral headache, nasal or sinus congestion or pain, and serosanguinous nasal discharge. Fever is also common. Most patients are not seen during this initial stage of local nasal and sinus infection. Two-thirds or more have more widespread infection and are lethargic or unconscious by the time of their first examination.

The infection often spreads into the palate, resulting in a black necrotic lesion. This is an important diagnostic sign. Necrotic lesions may also be found on the nasal mucosa. Nasal septum or palatal perforation is frequent.

If the infection spreads into the orbit, periorbital or perinasal swelling will occur and progress to induration and discoloration. Ptosis, proptosis, dilation and fixation of the pupil, and loss of vision may occur. Drainage of black pus from the eye is a useful diagnostic sign. From the orbit infection may spread into the brain leading to frontal lobe necrosis and abscess formation.

Examination of the cerebrospinal fluid (CSF) is seldom helpful. The protein concentration may be slightly raised, but the glucose concentration is usually normal. There may be a modest mononuclear pleocytosis. CSF cultures are sterile.

Computed tomographic (CT) and magnetic resonance imaging (MRI) scans are helpful in defining the extent of bone and soft-tissue destruction, but are more useful in planning surgical intervention than in establishing a diagnosis. CT scans of the head often reveal sinus opacification, but other changes are minimal, even when there is massive orbital infection. MRI scanning may be preferred for the diabetic patient for whom CT contrast agents may be contraindicated.

13.4.2 Pulmonary mucormycosis

This condition is seldom diagnosed during life. Mucormycosis may develop in the lungs as a result of aspiration of infectious material, or following inhalation, or from haematogenous or lymphatic spread during dissemination. Most cases occur in neutropenic cancer patients undergoing remission induction treatment. If untreated, haematogenous dissemination to other organs, particularly the brain, will often occur. The infection is fatal within 2–3 weeks.

The most common presentation in a neutropenic cancer patient is an unremitting fever (greater than 38°C) that fails to respond to broad-spectrum antibacterial treatment. Cough is a common presenting symptom. Haemoptysis and pleuritic chest pain are uncommon, but when present are helpful in suggesting a fungal infection. However, there are no characteristic symptoms or clinical signs to distinguish mucormycosis from aspergillosis (see Chapter 10).

The radiological signs are also non-specific, but infiltrates and nodules are more frequent than consolidation or cavitation. Pleural effusion is uncommon.

13.4.3 Gastrointestinal mucormycosis

This is an uncommon condition that has usually been encountered in malnourished infants or children. Lesions are most common in the stomach, colon and ileum. It is seldom diagnosed during life.

The symptoms are varied and depend on the site affected. Non-specific abdominal pain and haematemesis are typical. Necrotic ulcers develop and peritonitis follows if intestinal perforation occurs. Intestinal mucormycosis is a fulminant illness ending in death within several weeks due to bowel infarction, sepsis or haemorrhagic shock.

13.4.4 Cutaneous mucormycosis

This is a particular problem in patients with burns in whom spread to underlying tissue is common. The initial signs include fever, swelling and changes in the appearance of the burn wound. The development of severe underlying necrosis and infarction in a burn should suggest the diagnosis.

Mucormycotic gangrenous cellulitis can follow other forms of trauma to the skin. In diabetic or immunosuppressed patients, cutaneous lesions may arise at an insulin injection site or a catheter insertion site. Necrotizing cutaneous mucormycosis has also occurred in patients who have had contaminated surgical dressings or splints applied to their skin.

Cutaneous lesions resembling ecthyma gangrenosum may develop following haematogenous dissemination of the fungus in immunosuppressed patients. The lesions begin as an erythematous, indurated painful cellulitis, then evolve into ulcers covered with a black eschar.

13.4.5 Disseminated mucormycosis

This may follow any of the four forms of mucormycosis described so far, but it is usually seen in neutropenic patients with a pulmonary infection. Less commonly, dissemination occurs from the gastrointestinal tract, burns or other cutaneous lesions. The most common site of spread is the brain, but metastatic necrotic lesions have also been found in the spleen, heart and other organs. Disseminated mucormycosis is seldom diagnosed during life, but occasional patients develop metastatic cutaneous lesions which permit an earlier diagnosis.

Cerebral infection following haematogenous dissemination is distinct from the rhinocerebral form of mucormycosis. The lesions often lead to focal neurological signs. The diagnosis is difficult, but should be considered in a neutropenic patient who becomes confused, obtunded or somnolent. CT and MRI scans are useful in locating the lesions, but the findings are non-specific. Investigation of the CSF is unhelpful: protein, glucose and cell abnormalities are non-specific and cultures are sterile.

13.4.6   Other forms of mucormycosis

Isolated mucormycotic brain lesions have been reported in parenteral drug abusers. Other unusual focal forms of mucormycosis include endocarditis, osteomyelitis and pyelonephritis.

13.5   **Differential diagnosis**

Rhinocerebral mucormycosis is a dramatic and distinctive condition, but it can be confused with cavernous sinus thrombosis, bacterial orbital cellulitis or rhinocerebral aspergillosis or hyalohyphomycosis.

The clinical manifestations of pulmonary mucormycosis cannot be distinguished from Gram-negative bacterial pneumonia, aspergillosis or hyalohyphomycosis.

13.6   **Essential investigations and their interpretation**

Because mucormycosis is such an aggressive infection, an early diagnosis is essential for successful treatment. It is, however, often difficult to obtain.

13.6.1   Microscopy

The microscopic demonstration of Mucorales in clinical material taken from necrotic lesions, or in sputum or bronchoalveolar lavage (BAL) fluid is more significant than their isolation in culture. These organisms can be distinguished from other moulds, such as *Aspergillus* species, due to their characteristic broad, non-septate filaments with right-angled branching.

13.6.2   Culture

Nasal, palatal and sputum cultures are seldom helpful, but specimens should be sent for culture if the clinician suspects mucormycosis. Because the Mucorales are common contaminants, isolation of these organisms from material obtained from a necrotic lesion, or from sputum or BAL fluid must be interpreted with caution. However, if the patient is diabetic or immunosuppressed, the isolation should not be ignored.

13.6.3   Serological tests

There are no routine serological tests for mucormycosis available at present.

13.7   **Management**

If treatment of mucormycosis is to be successful, underlying disorders must be controlled, infected necrotic tissue must be removed, and amphotericin B must be administered. Other antifungal drugs have no role in the management of this infection.

Management of rhinocerebral infection in the diabetic patient should consist of prompt correction of acidosis, rapid surgical debridement of infected and necrotic tissue, and administration of amphotericin B. The drug is used at a dosage of at least 1.0 mg/kg per day and should be continued for 8–10 weeks.

In neutropenic and other immunosuppressed patients with mucormycosis, amphotericin B should be given at a dosage of 1.0–1.5 mg/kg per day from the outset as there is no time for gradual escalation (see Chapter 3). Immuno-suppressive drugs should be reduced in dose or discontinued if this will not harm the patient.

If mucormycosis fails to respond to high doses of the conventional formulation of amphotericin B, most clinicians now change to one of the lipid-based formulations of the drug at dosages of 3–5 mg/kg or higher and continue this until the patient recovers, or for at least 2 weeks before reverting to conventional amphotericin B. Administration of lipid-based amphotericin B is also recommended for patients in whom the conventional formulation is contraindicated because of renal impairment, or who develop side-effects that would otherwise necessitate discontinuation of the drug. It remains unclear as to whether these new formulations differ from each other in terms of clinical benefit in mucormycosis.

If a patient with mucormycosis confined to one region of the lung does not respond to amphotericin B treatment within 48–72 h, surgical resection should be considered. Although a wedge resection is sometimes sufficient, complete lobar or segmental resection is often required. The more widespread the infection is, the less beneficial the surgical intervention.

In individuals with cutaneous mucormycosis, aggressive surgical debridement of the necrotic lesions and surrounding infected tissue is the single most important component of treatment. Administration of amphotericin B is also advised. Skin grafting is often required to repair the defects remaining after debridement.

The optimum duration and total dose of amphotericin B that should be given to patients with mucormycosis has not been determined. Treatment must be individualized according to the patient's clinical response and the rate of clearing of the infection. In most reports a total dose of at least 2 g of amphotericin B has been given, although some patients have received as much as 4 g. With prompt diagnosis and treatment, up to 50% of diabetic patients with rhinocerebral mucormycosis can be cured. In neutropenic cancer patients the prognosis is poor if the neutrophil count does not recover.

14   Blastomycosis

14.1   Definition

The term blastomycosis is used to refer to infections due to the dimorphic fungus *Blastomyces dermatitidis*. Following inhalation this organism can cause pulmonary infection in normal individuals, but it often spreads to involve other organs, in particular the skin and bones.

14.2   Geographical distribution

Most cases of blastomycosis have been reported from the mid-western and southeastern regions of North America, but the disease also occurs in Central and South America and parts of Africa.

14.3   The causal organism and its habitat

B. dermatitidis is a dimorphic fungus. It exists in nature as mycelium and as large, round budding cells in infected tissue.

It appears that the natural habitat of *B. dermatitidis* is the soil, although attempts to recover it have seldom proved successful. The fungus appears to survive best in moist soil containing organic debris or in rotting wood.

Unlike histoplasmosis and coccidioidomycosis, there is no accepted means of identifying subclinical and resolved infection in the human population and this has also hindered attempts to delineate the endemic regions. Apart from epidemics, blastomycosis is much more common in men than women or children. It often occurs in individuals with an outdoor occupation or recreational interest.

14.4   Clinical manifestations

Infection follows inhalation of *B. dermatitidis* spores that have been released into the air. The lungs are the usual initial site of infection. In some cases the infection will resolve without dissemination to other organs, but in others it spreads to involve the skin, bone, prostate or other organs. Risk factors for disseminated infection have not been identified.

167

14.4.1   **Pulmonary blastomycosis**

Up to 50% of individuals develop no symptoms following inhalation of *B. dermatitidis* spores and their lung lesion is not detected until the infection has spread to other organs. Of the remainder, some develop an acute symptomatic pulmonary infection, similar to that seen with histoplasmosis or coccidioidomycosis, and others develop a chronic progressive pulmonary infection.

Patients with acute pulmonary blastomycosis develop a flu-like illness. The most common symptoms are fever, chills, productive cough, myalgia, arthralgia and pleuritic chest pain. The radiological findings are non-specific and include lobar or segmental consolidation, often in the lower lobes. Most patients recover after 2–12 weeks of symptoms, but some return months later with infection of other sites. Other patients with acute blastomycosis fail to recover and develop a chronic pulmonary infection or disseminated infection.

The symptoms of chronic pulmonary blastomycosis are similar to those of tuberculosis and include productive cough, haemoptysis, weight loss, night sweats, malaise and fever that is often low grade. Spontaneous resolution of the infection is unusual. The radiological findings are more dramatic than those seen in patients with acute infection and include consolidation, fibronodular infiltrates, mass-like lesions, diffuse infiltrates, pleural thickening, and pleural effusions. Cavitation is uncommon.

14.4.2   **Cutaneous blastomycosis**

Haematogenous spread gives rise to cutaneous lesions in over 70% of patients with disseminated blastomycosis. These tend to be painless and present either as raised verrucous lesions with irregular borders, or as ulcers. The face, upper limbs, neck and scalp are the most frequent sites of involvement. Cutaneous lesions sometimes develop from lesions in underlying bone.

14.4.3   **Osteoarticular blastomycosis**

Osteomyelitis occurs in about 30% of patients with disseminated blastomycosis. The spine, ribs and long bones are the most common sites of infection. The lesions often remain asymptomatic until the infection spreads into contiguous joints, or into adjacent soft tissue causing abscess formation

and sinus tract development. Infection of the spine can involve adjacent vertebral bodies with destruction of the intervening disc space.

The radiological findings are not specific and the well-defined osteolytic or osteoblastic lesions cannot be distinguished from those of other fungal or bacterial infections. Periosteal proliferation is unusual.

Arthritis is less common than osteomyelitis, occurring in up to 10% of patients with blastomycosis either as a result of haematogenous dissemination from the lung, or spread from a contiguous bone lesion. The most common sites of infection are the knee, ankle, elbow and wrist. The symptoms include swelling, pain and limited movement in the affected joint.

14.4.4 Genitourinary blastomycosis

The prostate, epididymis or testis are involved in 15–35% of men with disseminated blastomycosis. The prostate may be tender and enlarged, resulting in obstruction. Epididymitis presents as scrotal swelling with or without a draining sinus. Infection often spreads to the adjacent testis.

On occasion, venereal transmission of *B. dermatitidis* infection has resulted in self-limited genital ulceration or endometrial infection in the woman.

14.4.5 Other forms of disseminated blastomycosis

Haematogenous spread of infection to the brain has been reported in occasional patients with disseminated blastomycosis. Manifestations of central nervous system (CNS) infection include meningitis and spinal or brain abscess formation. Meningitis is indolent in onset and tends to occur late in the course of *B. dermatitidis* infection. It is often lethal and is indistinguishable from other forms of chronic meningitis such as tuberculosis or cryptococcosis.

Other organs, such as the adrenal glands or liver are sometimes involved. Choroiditis and endophthalmitis have been reported.

14.5 Blastomycosis in special hosts

Although blastomycosis has been reported in patients with impaired T-cell mediated immunological function, it is much less common than histoplasmosis or coccidioidomycosis. Occasional patients with acquired immunodeficiency syndrome (AIDS) have developed fulminant blastomycosis with widespread dissemination following endogenous reactivation of previous infection.

14.6 Differential diagnosis

Tuberculosis of the lung, skin, bone or genital tract, coccidioidomycosis of the lung, bone or meninges, and mucocutaneous paracoccidioidomycosis are other infections that can be confused with blastomycosis. However, the endemic regions for blastomycosis have almost no overlap with those of the other two fungal infections.

14.7 Essential investigations and their interpretation

14.7.1 Microscopy

Microscopic examination of wet preparations of pus, sputum, bronchial washings, urine or other clinical material can permit the diagnosis of blastomycosis if the characteristic large round cells with thick refractile walls and broad-based single buds are seen. Atypical *B. dermatitidis* cells can, however, be confused with other pathogens, such as single or non-budding cells of *Paracoccidioides brasiliensis*, *Histoplasma capsulatum* var. *duboisii*, and non-encapsulated cells of *Cryptococcus neoformans*.

14.7.2 Culture

The definitive diagnosis of blastomycosis depends on isolation of the fungus in culture. Identifiable mycelial colonies can be obtained after incubation at 25–30°C for 1–3 weeks, but cultures should be retained for 4 weeks before being discarded. The small round single-celled spores are borne on simple lateral conidiophores. Subculture of the mycelial isolate on brain–heart infusion agar or blood–glucose–cysteine agar at 37°C should result in the production of the unicellular form, confirming the identification. If a more rapid identification (24 h) is desired, the initial mycelial culture can be subjected to an exoantigen test.

In culture at 25–30°C, African strains of *B. dermatitidis* produce more spores than North American strains; at 37°C African strains produce chain-like clusters of cells. In addition, antigen A, which gives more specific results in serological tests, is absent from African strains.

14.7.3   Serological tests

Serological methods are of limited usefulness in the diagnosis of blastomycosis because of the high incidence of false-positive and false-negative reactions. The complement fixation test with unpurified antigen has been the least sensitive and least specific method. The immunodiffusion (ID) test is more specific, but negative reactions have been obtained in 10% of patients with disseminated infection and over 60% with localized infection. However, a positive reaction in the ID test can be considered diagnostic for blastomycosis.

14.8   **Management**

Many patients with acute pulmonary blastomycosis are asymptomatic and recover without treatment. However, some later develop serious complications. For this reason, patients with asymptomatic infection who are left untreated should be monitored for signs of reactivation. All patients with symptomatic infection require treatment.

Oral itraconazole is the drug of choice for non-immuno-compromised patients with indolent forms of blastomycosis. It should be given at a dosage of 200 mg/day for up to 6 months, or for at least 3 months after the lesions have resolved. If there is no obvious improvement, or if there are signs of progression, the dose should be increased to 400 mg/day. Oral ketoconazole is almost as effective, but less well tolerated than itraconazole. Treatment is usually initiated at a dosage of 400 mg/day, increasing to 600 mg and then 800 mg as required. Fluconazole is less effective than itraconazole or ketoconazole but it is sometimes useful in patients who do not tolerate or cannot absorb itraconazole or ketoconazole. The minimum dosage should be 400–800 mg/day.

Amphotericin B remains the drug of choice for patients with life-threatening infection and those with CNS involvement. It should also be used in immunocompromised patients and those who have failed to respond to azole treatment. The recommended dose is 0.3–0.6 mg/kg per day (or 0.6–0.8 mg/kg on alternate days) to a total dose of 1.5–2.5 g. Lower doses are associated with an increased risk of relapse. Patients who respond to initial treatment with amphotericin B can often be changed to itraconazole for the remainder of their treatment.

15   Coccidioidomycosis

15.1   Definition

The term coccidioidomycosis is used to refer to infections due to the dimorphic fungus *Coccidioides immitis*. Following inhalation, this organism tends to cause a mild and transient pulmonary infection in normal individuals, but it can proceed to cause progressive infection of the lungs or more generalized infection.

15.2   Geographical distribution

Most cases of coccidioidomycosis have been reported from the southwestern USA, and parts of Central and South America. However, the infection has also been diagnosed outside these regions among individuals who had earlier resided in or visited an endemic region.

15.3   The causal organism and its habitat

C. immitis is a dimorphic fungus. It exists in nature as a mycelium which fragments into arthrospores. In tissue, it forms characteristic large round thick-walled spherules which contain large numbers of endospores. Mycelium is seldom produced in tissue, but is sometimes found in chronic lung lesions.

C. immitis is a soil-inhabiting fungus with a restricted geographical distribution. It is confined to certain hot, arid parts of the southwestern USA, and parts of Central and South America. Climatic conditions in these regions consist of a season of rainfall which favours mycelial proliferation in the soil and a long hot summer period during which large numbers of arthrospores are produced and dispersed in dust in the air. Dust storms often spread the organism far outside its endemic regions.

It is estimated that 50 000–100 000 persons are infected per annum in the USA. In certain endemic parts of North America, skin testing has demonstrated that more than 90% of the population have had the infection.

15.4	**Clinical manifestations**

In most individuals inhalation of C. *immitis* arthrospores leads to a mild and transient pulmonary infection which resolves without treatment. In immunosuppressed or other predisposed individuals, the infection can cause chronic pulmonary infection or more widespread disease. This is usually fatal if left untreated.

15.4.1	Primary pulmonary coccidioidomycosis

About 60% of newly infected persons develop no symptoms following inhalation of C. *immitis* arthrospores. The remainder develop symptoms after an incubation period of 1–4 weeks. Higher levels of exposure to dust containing arthrospores are associated with an increased likelihood of acute symptomatic disease.

Most symptomatic patients develop a mild or moderate flu-like illness that resolves without treatment. The symptoms include fever, chest pain, cough, malaise, chills, night sweats, arthralgia and loss of appetite. Up to 50% of patients develop a mild, diffuse erythematous or maculopapular rash, covering the trunk and limbs, within the first few days of the onset of symptoms. More dramatic and persistent is the rash of erythema nodosum or erythema multiforme which occur in up to 30% of infected persons, but are more common in women. These signs occur up to 3 weeks after symptoms first appear and resolve over several weeks. Both are often accompanied by arthralgia in one or more joints.

The most common radiological finding is segmental pneumonia which is seen in about 50% of cases. About 30% of infected individuals show minimal infiltrates, but 20% develop enlarged hilar lymph nodes or a pleural effusion. In addition, single or multiple nodules, as well as thick- or thin-walled cavities and enlarged mediastinal lymph nodes can occur. In most cases, the radiological abnormalities resolve in 1–3 weeks.

15.4.2	Chronic pulmonary coccidioidomycosis

About 5% of infected individuals are left with residual signs of pulmonary coccidioidomycosis. In some cases, solid nodules are formed in the infiltrate. These are benign. In others, persistent thin-walled cavities develop. These often disappear within 2 years. Most patients are asymptomatic, but haemoptysis occurs in 25% of cases. Onset of fever, chest pain and dyspnoea is a sign that residual lung cavities have enlarged and ruptured into the pleural space causing a bronchopleural fistula or empyema.

In immunosuppressed patients with coccidioidomycosis, symptoms often persist and the patient can remain ill for months with fever, cough, chest pain and prostration. This acute progressive pneumonia can be fatal, often without disseminated infection.

Chronic progressive pneumonia can occur in patients who are not debilitated or immunosuppressed. This illness mimics tuberculosis. The symptoms include fever, cough, chest pain and weight loss. These patients have apical fibronodular lesions with small cavities.

15.4.3 Disseminated coccidioidomycosis

Fewer than 1% of infected individuals develop disseminated coccidioidomycosis. This is a progressive, often fatal illness that tends to occur in immunosuppressed or debilitated individuals. Men are five times more susceptible to dissemination than women, but the ratio is reversed if the woman is pregnant. Infants and members of certain non-Caucasian racial groups are also more susceptible to disseminated infection.

In most cases, disseminated coccidioidomycosis develops within 12 months of the initial infection, although it can occur much later following reactivation of a quiescent infection in an immunosuppressed individual. Many cases of disseminated coccidioidomycosis in patients with the acquired immune deficiency syndrome (AIDS) have been due to reactivation.

The clinical manifestations of disseminated coccidioidomycosis range from a fulminant illness that is fatal within a few weeks if left untreated, to an indolent chronic illness that persists for months or years. One or more sites may be involved, but cutaneous, soft-tissue, bone, joint and meningeal infection is most common.

In immunosuppressed individuals, widespread rapid dissemination often occurs. Patients present with dramatic sweats, dyspnoea at rest, fever and weight loss. In most cases, chest radiographs reveal diffuse, miliary lesions. Patients undergo rapid clinical deterioration and die if left untreated.

Cutaneous and subcutaneous lesions are among the most common manifestations of disseminated coccidioidomycosis. Cutaneous lesions may be single or multiple and can persist for long periods. Their appearance is varied: verrucous papules, erythematous plaques and nodules have been described. Underlying bone or joint lesions may be found.

Osteomyelitis occurs in about 40% of patients with disseminated coccidioidomycosis. The spine, ribs, cranial bones and ends of the long bones are the most common sites of infection. Patients often remain asymptomatic, but persistent dull pain may occur. Irregular lytic or sclerotic lesions are seen on radiographs. Computed tomographic (CT) scans are useful in detecting asymptomatic lesions and should be performed in all patients with serious or disseminated infection. The infection may spread into contiguous joints causing arthritis, or into adjacent soft tissue, causing subcutaneous abscess formation. Draining sinuses often appear. The ankles and knees are the most common sites of joint infection.

Meningitis is the most serious complication of coccidioidomycosis. It occurs in 30–50% of patients with disseminated infection. It often gives rise to hydrocephalus and is fatal if left untreated. The symptoms are non-specific and insidious in onset. Persistent headache is often the earliest symptom. Mental changes, such as drowsiness and confusion, also occur. Other symptoms include loss of appetite, nausea and weight loss. Fever is minimal or absent in indolent cases. CT scans of the head are abnormal in most patients, the most common finding being ventricular enlargement.

Most patients with symptomatic meningitis have abnormal cerebrospinal fluid (CSF) findings, including an elevated protein concentration, a lowered glucose concentration and a lymphocytic pleocytosis.

Other sites of infection include lymph nodes, liver, spleen and adrenal gland. Chorioretinitis, peritonitis, prostatitis and epididymitis are among the other unusual manifestations that have been reported.

15.5 Coccidioidomycosis in special hosts

15.5.1 Patients with AIDS

Coccidioidomycosis has become a serious problem in patients with AIDS who have resided in, or travelled through endemic regions. Most cases among patients with AIDS living in endemic regions are recently acquired and not due to reactivation of latent infection. However, in a small number of cases, a previously acquired infection is reactivated and the disease develops while the patient is living outside the endemic regions.

Most patients with AIDS with coccidioidomycosis present with pulmonary disease. In many, chest radiographs reveal diffuse reticulonodular infiltrates. About 70% of these individuals die within 1 month despite antifungal treatment. Skin, soft-tissue, bone, joint and meningeal infection is less common in patients with AIDS with disseminated coccidioidomycosis than in other patients.

15.6 Differential diagnosis

The clinical presentation of primary pulmonary coccidioidomycosis is similar to that of blastomycosis and histoplasmosis. The symptoms and clinical signs of chronic meningeal coccidioidomycosis are similar to those of cryptococcosis.

The large, cold abscesses that develop in soft tissue adjacent to *C. immitis* bone lesions can be mistaken for tuberculosis.

The radiological presentation in patients with residual lung cavities due to *C. immitis* infection is similar to that of a number of other infectious and non-infectious conditions, including cryptococcosis, tuberculosis and bacterial lung abscess. In most of these other conditions the cavities have a thicker wall, or more extensive surrounding infiltrate. The diffuse lung infiltrates that are found in patients with AIDS with coccidioidomycosis can be confused with *Pneumocystis carinii* infection.

15.7 Essential investigations and their interpretation

It is essential to inform the laboratory if a diagnosis of coccidioidomycosis is suspected, to ensure that proper precautions in handling of specimens and cultures are observed.

15.7.1 Microscopy

Microscopic examination of wet preparations of clinical material, such as sputum, joint fluid, pus or sediment of centrifuged CSF specimens, can permit the diagnosis of coccidioidomycosis if the characteristic large, thick-walled endospore-containing spherules are seen. Immature spherules and liberated endospores can, however, be confused with other pathogens, such as non-budding cells of *Blastomyces dermatitidis* or *Cryptococcus neoformans*. In general, spherules are easier to detect in pus, sputum or joint fluid than in blood or CSF.

15.7.2 Culture

The organism can be isolated from sputum, joint fluid, CSF sediment, pus and other specimens. Cultures must be set up in secure containers (slopes rather than plates) and handled with great care because of the danger of infection from the large concentrations of easily dispersed and highly infectious arthrospores. Identifiable mycelial colonies can be obtained after incubation at 25–30°C for 2–7 days, but cultures should be retained for at least 3 weeks before being discarded.

In culture, *C. immitis* must be distinguished from other moulds that produce arthrospores. The exoantigen test permits rapid identification. It is also useful for identifying atypical *C. immitis* isolates that fail to form arthrospores.

15.7.3 Skin tests

A positive coccidioidin or spherulin skin test result does not distinguish present from past infection. Conversion from a negative to a positive result is a sign of recent infection, because it occurs within 4 weeks of the onset of symptoms in 90–95% of patients. False-negative results are common in anergic patients with disseminated coccidioidomycosis. Unlike the histoplasmin skin test (see Chapter 16), coccidioidin does not interfere with the results of subsequent serological tests.

15.7.4 Serological tests

Serological tests are helpful in the diagnosis of coccidioidomycosis, although occasional cross-reactions occur in patients with histoplasmosis or blastomycosis.

Tests for the detection of IgM antibodies against *C. immitis* are most useful for diagnosing acute infection. These antibodies can be detected in most patients within 4 weeks of the onset of infection, but disappear within 2–6 months, even if the patient develops a disseminated infection. IgG antibodies are most useful for detecting the later stages of coccidioidomycosis. These antibodies do not appear until 4–12 weeks after infection. In disseminated infection, IgG antibodies persist until death or until the patient recovers. The IgM titre is not significant, but IgG titres rise with progression of the infection and decline as the patient improves.

IgM antibodies can be detected with the latex particle agglutination (LPA) test, tube precipitin (TP) test or immunodiffusion (ID) test. The LPA test is more sensitive, faster and simpler than the classical TP test, but gives at least 10% of false-positive reactions with serum and CSF specimens. For this reason a positive LPA test result must be confirmed with other methods. The ID test with heated coccidioidin as antigen has replaced the TP test as the method of choice for diagnosing acute infection. It is more sensitive, faster and simpler than the TP method. Although uncommon, a positive ID reaction with CSF is an indication of meningitis.

IgG antibodies can be detected with the classical CF test or using ID tests with filtered coccidioidin as antigen. In general, a rising CF titre (greater than 1 : 16) is consistent with spread of infection from the lungs. More than 50% of patients with disseminated infection have titres of more than 1 : 16. CF titres of 1 : 4 or 1 : 8 should not be considered as significant unless confirmed with a positive ID result.

The detection of antibodies in CSF is indicative of meningitis and remains the single most useful diagnostic test for that condition.

Serological tests can be useful in the diagnosis of coccidioidomycosis in patients with AIDS although they are more likely to have negative results than other infected individuals. Conversely, a positive CF result in a human immunodeficiency virus (HIV)-infected patient, even in the absence of clinical illness, predicts impending disease.

15.8 Management
15.8.1 Primary pulmonary coccidioidomycosis

Most newly infected individuals have an uncomplicated, self-limited illness and recover without antifungal treatment. No antifungal agent has been shown to shorten the course of the illness or to reduce the likelihood of later complications.

Therefore it is reasonable to refrain from treatment if the illness appears to be following a benign course.

Fewer than 5% of all newly infected patients require treatment. Those who should be treated to prevent progression or dissemination of infection include infants, pregnant women, debilitated or immunosuppressed individuals, and members of high-risk racial groups.

Antifungal treatment is also indicated in non-compromised patients with persistent symptoms lasting for more than 6 weeks, persistent debilitation, extensive or progressive pulmonary involvement, persistent hilar or mediastinal lymph node enlargement, rising or elevated titres (greater than 1 : 16) of IgG antibodies, or negative skin test reactions.

The traditional treatment of choice in patients who require active management is amphotericin B. The usual regimen is 0.4–0.6 mg/kg per day. Provided the patient has stabilized, 0.8–1.0 mg/kg can be given at 48-h intervals. It is usually recommended that treatment is continued until a total dose of 0.5–1.5 g has been given.

With the advent of non-toxic oral antifungal agents, such as itraconazole and fluconazole, more clinicians are now treating patients with milder infections. The usual dose of itraconazole and fluconazole is 400 mg/day for 2–6 months. Oral ketoconazole (400 mg/day) can also be used, but is less well tolerated.

15.8.2 Chronic pulmonary coccidioidomycosis

Patients with small, asymptomatic cavities do not require treatment, but should be observed until spontaneous resolution occurs. Those with enlarging cavities often require surgical resection. This is indicated if the cavities are near the pleural surface, or if serious and persistent haemoptysis, or bacterial superinfection is a problem. It is advisable to give a short 4-week course of amphotericin B (0.4–0.6 mg/kg per day), commencing about 2 weeks before the surgical procedure.

Patients with chronic progressive pneumonia present a difficult problem. Treatment with amphotericin B (0.4–0.6 mg/kg per day) often arrests progression, but relapse is common after the drug is discontinued.

The results of a recent clinical trial suggest that fluconazole (200–400 mg/day) is an effective and well-tolerated treatment for chronic pulmonary coccidioidomycosis. However, the relapse rate is quite high when the drug is discontinued.

15.8.3   **Disseminated coccidioidomycosis**
The drug of choice for patients with non-meningeal disseminated coccidioidomycosis is amphotericin B. The usual adult dose is 1.0–1.5 mg/kg per day. Treatment should be continued until a total dose of 2.5–3.0 g has been given. The results of treatment are often disappointing and relapse is a common problem.

Both itraconazole (400 mg/day) and ketoconazole (400 mg/day) have been used to treat disseminated coccidioidomycosis, but the former is better tolerated. Fluconazole (400 mg/day) also appears to be effective in patients with cutaneous, soft-tissue, bone or joint lesions. However, long periods of treatment are often required and the relapse rate after discontinuing treatment is quite high.

Surgical debridement of infected tissue is important in the management of osteomyelitis and in the diagnosis and drainage of soft-tissue lesions.

Amphotericin B (1.0–1.5 mg/kg per day) is the most appropriate initial treatment for patients with AIDS with diffuse pneumonia. The drug should be continued until a total dose of 1.0 g has been given. Thereafter, itraconazole (400 mg/day) or fluconazole (400 mg/day) may be substituted if the patient has improved. Patients with AIDS with less severe forms of disseminated coccidioidomycosis, such as cutaneous or osteoarticular infection, can be treated with itraconazole or fluconazole from the outset.

15.8.4   **Meningitis**
Until the advent of oral treatment with fluconazole or itraconazole, the management of this serious form of coccidioidomycosis consisted of prolonged courses of intrathecal treatment with amphotericin B. This was associated with a high incidence of side-effects and complications. Recent clinical trials have demonstrated that fluconazole treatment (400 mg/day) leads to clinical improvement in up to 80% of patients. The response rate in patients with AIDS is lower. Treatment with fluconazole does not eradicate meningeal infection with *C. immitis* and the drug must be continued for life to prevent relapse.

However, because fluconazole is so much more benign than intrathecal amphotericin B, it is now the drug of choice for coccidioidal meningitis.

Itraconazole (400 mg/day) has also been used to treat this infection, but supportive evidence from large clinical trials is not available.

16   Histoplasmosis

16.1   Definition

The term histoplasmosis is used to refer to infections due to the dimorphic fungus *Histoplasma capsulatum*. Following inhalation, this organism tends to cause a mild and transient pulmonary infection in normal individuals, but it can proceed to cause chronic infection of the lungs or more widespread infection in predisposed patients.

16.2   Geographical distribution

Although histoplasmosis has a global distribution, it is most prevalent in the central region of North America and in Central and South America. Other endemic regions include Africa, Australia and parts of East Asia, in particular India and Malaysia.

16.3   The causal organism and its habitat

H. capsulatum is a dimorphic fungus. It exists in nature as a mycelium. In tissue it forms small round budding cells.

Two varieties of *H. capsulatum* are recognized: var. *capsulatum* and var. *duboisii*. The two varieties are indistinguishable in their mycelial (saprotrophic) forms, but differ in their parasitic forms. The cells of the tissue form of var. *duboisii* are much larger and have thicker walls than those of var. *capsulatum*.

The natural habitat of *H. capsulatum* is soil enriched with bird or bat droppings. If contaminated soil or bird roosts are disturbed during building construction or demolition, this can lead to enormous numbers of spores being dispersed in the air and result in large numbers of individuals being infected. Numerous epidemic outbreaks of histoplasmosis have been reported from the USA. Bat-roosting sites, such as caves, are also important sources of *H. capsulatum*, particularly in the tropics.

It is estimated that 500 000 persons are infected per annum in the USA, making it the most common endemic mycosis. In certain endemic parts of the USA, histoplasmin skin testing has demonstrated that more than 80% of the population have had the infection.

Although infections due to *H. capsulatum* var. *duboisii* have been confined to the central region of the African continent (and termed African histoplasmosis), infections with var. *capsulatum* have also been reported from parts of that continent.

16.4   Clinical manifestations

In most persons, inhalation of *H. capsulatum* spores leads to a transient pulmonary infection which subsides without treatment. In some predisposed individuals, however, the organism can cause chronic pulmonary infection or more widespread disease. This is a progressive, often fatal, illness.

16.4.1   Acute pulmonary histoplasmosis

Most normal individuals develop no symptoms following inhalation of low levels of *H. capsulatum* spores. Higher levels of exposure result in an acute symptomatic and often severe infection after an incubation period of 1–3 weeks.

Most symptomatic patients develop a non-specific flu-like illness that resolves without treatment. The most common symptoms are fever, chills, headache, myalgia, loss of appetite, cough and chest pain. About 10% of patients present with an aseptic arthritis or arthralgia associated with erythema multiforme or nodosum. Most otherwise normal persons will recover without treatment, their symptoms disappearing within 1–3 weeks. However, fatigue and weakness can persist for several months.

Chest radiographs are normal in most patients, but sometimes reveal small scattered nodular infiltrates. Hilar lymph node enlargement is often evident and pleural effusion may be found. The infiltrates tend to heal over several months leaving scattered calcifications throughout both lung fields. Healing of a localized infiltrate may result in the development of a residual round nodule, often termed a histoplasmoma, that enlarges as fibrous material is deposited around the lesion. If calcification is absent, these benign lesions cannot be distinguished from a neoplasm on chest radiographs.

Individuals reinfected with *H. capsulatum* develop a similar illness, but this is milder and occurs after a much shorter incubation period (less than 1 week). These patients present with abrupt onset of malaise, headache, chills, fever and cough, but the symptoms are less severe and of shorter duration. The radiological signs are different from those seen in newly infected individuals. Multiple small interstitial miliary nodules are present, but there is no mediastinal lymph node enlargement and pleural effusions are not seen. Late calcification does not occur. The illness tends to resolve without treatment.

Following inhalation of *H. capsulatum*, the organism gains access to the alveolar and interstitial lung tissue and then spreads through the lymphatics to the lymph nodes. In some patients this process results in mediastinal lymph node enlargement which in turn can lead to tracheal, bronchial or oesophageal obstruction. Mediastinal lymphadenitis undergoes spontaneous resolution in most patients.

16.4.2   **Chronic pulmonary histoplasmosis**

This slowly progressive illness usually occurs in middle-aged men with underlying chronic obstructive lung disease. It first manifests itself as a transient, segmental pneumonia that sometimes heals without treatment, but often progresses to fibrosis and cavitation with destruction of significant amounts of lung tissue. If left untreated, death can result from progressive lung failure.

In patients with pneumonia, the symptoms often include productive cough, fever, chills, weight loss, malaise, night sweats and pleuritic chest pain. The typical radiological findings in these patients are interstitial infiltrates in the apical segments of the upper lobes of the lung.

The most prominent symptoms in patients with chronic fibrosis and cavitation are cough and sputum production. Other symptoms include fever, chest pain, fatigue and weight loss. Haemoptysis develops in more than 30% of these individuals. Chest radiographs will reveal progressive cavitation and fibrosis. Cavities with walls thicker than 3 mm in diameter are associated with established and continuing infection. Lesions are more common in the right upper lobe than in the left, but bilateral lesions develop in about 25% of patients and, in time, the infection will spread to the lower lobes. Pleural effusion is uncommon, but pleural thickening adjacent to lesions is found in 50% of patients.

16.4.3   **Disseminated histoplasmosis**

This is a progressive, often lethal illness that has been estimated to occur in one in 2000 exposed individuals, in particular those with T-cell mediated immunological defects.

The clinical manifestations of disseminated histoplasmosis range from an acute illness that is fatal within a few weeks if left untreated (often seen in infants and immunosuppressed patients) to an indolent, chronic illness that can affect a wide range of sites. Treatment is essential for all patients with disseminated histoplasmosis.

In infants and immunosuppressed patients, acute disseminated histoplasmosis often presents as high fever, chills, prostration, malaise, loss of appetite and weight loss. The liver and spleen are enlarged and liver function tests are abnormal. Anaemia is common. Chest radiographs are often normal, but if abnormal, diffuse interstitial infiltrates are more common than focal infiltrates. Pleural effusions are uncommon. Mucosal lesions can occur, but are much less common than in patients with indolent progression of the illness.

In non-immunosuppressed individuals, disseminated histoplasmosis follows an indolent, chronic course. Often chest radiographs are normal. Hepatic infection is common, but enlargement of the liver and spleen is not as pronounced as in patients with fulminant infection. Adrenal gland destruction is a common problem. Mucosal ulcers are found in over 60% of patients with indolent infection. The mouth and throat are often affected, but lesions also occur on the lip, nose, glans penis and other sites. Most patients have a single lesion, painless at first, with a characteristic, distinct heaped-up margin. Cutaneous lesions are uncommon, occurring in less than 10% of patients.

Meningitis is a chronic complication of histoplasmosis, occurring in 10–25% of patients with indolent disseminated infection. Headache is the most common presenting symptom: it is often mild. Most patients have abnormal cerebrospinal fluid (CSF) findings, including an elevated protein concentration, a lowered glucose concentration and a mild lymphocytic pleocytosis. *H. capsulatum* has been isolated from the CSF in 25–50% of cases.

Other manifestations of chronic disseminated histoplasmosis include endocarditis (often with large vegetations) and mucosal ulcerations in the gastrointestinal tract. Occasional cases of bone and joint infection have occurred in infants and children.

16.4.4 African histoplasmosis

The clinical manifestations of *H. capsulatum* var. *duboisii* infection differ in a number of respects from those of var. *capsulatum* infection described in the preceding sections. The illness is indolent in onset and the predominant sites affected are the skin and bones. Those with more widespread infection involving the liver, spleen and other organs have a febrile wasting illness that is fatal within weeks or months if left untreated.

Cutaneous lesions are common in patients with African histoplasmosis. Multiple papular lesions often develop on the face and trunk. Nodular lesions are less common. Both nodules and papules often enlarge and ulcerate. Osteomyelitis occurs in about 30% of patients with African histoplasmosis. The spine, ribs, cranial bones, sternum and long bones are the most common sites of infection and multiple lesions are often found. The lesions are often painless. The infection may spread into contiguous joints causing arthritis, or into adjacent soft tissue, causing a purulent subcutaneous abscess. Draining sinuses often appear.

16.5 Histoplasmosis in special hosts
16.5.1 Patients with AIDS

Histoplasmosis is an acquired immune deficiency syndrome (AIDS)-defining illness that occurs in 2–5% of patients with AIDS living in the endemic regions of the USA. The disease develops as the result of an acute infection or reactivation of an old latent infection. Up to 95% of patients with AIDS with histoplasmosis present with disseminated infection.

Most patients with AIDS with histoplasmosis present with non-specific symptoms, such as fever and weight loss, that are often gradual in onset. Up to 25% of patients have an enlarged liver and spleen and a similar proportion have anaemia, leucopenia and thrombocytopenia. Mucosal lesions are uncommon, but 15–20% of patients have an erythematous, maculopapular non-pruritic skin rash. About 30% of patients with AIDS with histoplasmosis have normal chest radiographs on admission, but 50% have diffuse interstitial infiltrates. Central nervous system (CNS) involvement occurs in 10–20% of cases: the manifestations include meningitis and focal brain lesions.

Ten to twenty per cent of patients with AIDS with histoplasmosis have presented with high fever, hypotension, hepatic and renal failure, respiratory distress and disseminated intravascular coagulation. This acute septic presentation appears to be a late manifestation of histoplasmosis in patients in whom the diagnosis has been missed. The death rate in these cases is high.

16.6 Differential diagnosis

The clinical presentation of acute pulmonary histoplasmosis is similar to that of many other conditions. The clinical and radiological presentation of chronic pulmonary histoplasmosis is similar to that of tuberculosis and coccidioidomycosis. The mucocutaneous lesions of chronic disseminated histoplasmosis can be confused with a number of other infectious and non-infectious conditions, including tuberculosis, syphilis, paracoccidioidomycosis and lichen planus.

16.7 Essential investigations and their interpretation

16.7.1 Microscopy

Microscopic examination of wet preparations of clinical material, such as sputum or pus, is not a suitable method for the diagnosis of histoplasmosis. All material should be examined as stained smears.

If microscopic examination of Wright-stained peripheral blood smears, or stained tissue sections, or other specimens from individuals who have resided in, or visited, endemic regions reveals small oval budding cells (often clustered within macrophages), the diagnosis of histoplasmosis should be suspected. *H. capsulatum* var. *capsulatum* cells can, however, be confused with other pathogens, such as *Penicillium marneffei*, as well as with atypical small cells of *Blastomyces dermatitidis* and small, non-encapsulated cells of *Cryptococcus neoformans*.

If clinical specimens contain large thick-walled cells and the patient has resided in or visited the African continent, *H. capsulatum* var. *duboisii* should be suspected as the pathogen.

Organisms tend to be much more abundant in peripheral blood smears and bronchial washings from patients with AIDS.

16.7.2 Culture

The definitive diagnosis of histoplasmosis depends on isolation of the fungus in culture. Incubation of cultures should be at 25–30°C for 4–6 weeks. It is often difficult to distinguish the mycelial colonies of *H. capsulatum* from those of *B. dermatitidis* and species of *Chrysosporium* and *Sepedonium*. Unequivocal identification of a mycelial isolate as *H. capsulatum* requires conversion to the yeast form which can take 3–6 weeks, or exoantigen testing which permits specific identification within 48–72 h.

H. capsulatum has been isolated from blood, sputum, bone marrow, pus, tissue and other specimens. Lysis-centrifugation has been the most useful method for recovering it from blood.

16.7.3 Skin tests

The histoplasmin skin test is not recommended for diagnosis of histoplasmosis, because a positive result does not distinguish present from past infection. Nor does a negative result rule out active infection. Moreover, it can induce the formation of antibodies making the results of subsequent serological tests difficult to interpret.

16.7.4 Serological tests

Serological tests are useful in the diagnosis of histoplasmosis. The immunodiffusion (ID) and complement fixation (CF) tests, with histoplasmin as antigen, are positive in about 80% of patients, including those with an acute self-limited infection. False-negative reactions can occur in immunosuppressed patients with disseminated histoplasmosis.

The CF test is more sensitive than ID in histoplasmosis. No more than 1% of patients with a negative CF test result will give a positive ID reaction. However, the CF test is not altogether specific and cross-reactions can occur in patients with blastomycosis or coccidioidomycosis. Nonspecific CF tests tend to give titres of 1:8–1:32. However, similar titres are often obtained in tests with serum from patients with proven histoplasmosis. CF titres of at least 1:32 or rising titres in serial specimens suggest active infection.

The ID test is more specific, but less sensitive than CF for histoplasmosis. Using histoplasmin as antigen, two major precipitin bands can be detected. The H band is specific for active histoplasmosis, but only occurs in 10–25% of patients. The M band can be detected in up to 85% of patients with active infection, but may also be found in patients with past infection, or in those who have had a recent histoplasmin skin test. Because the H and M bands are specific for histoplasmosis, the ID test provides a more specific diagnosis with serum specimens that have low CF titres or that cross-react in CF tests.

Antigen detection is the most useful serological method for diagnosis of disseminated histoplasmosis in patients with AIDS. *H. capsulatum* antigen has been detected in the blood of 85% and in the urine of 95% of these individuals. Antigen has also been detected in CSF and bronchoalveolar lavage fluid. Antigen levels in the urine fall in patients receiving antifungal treatment and rise in those who have relapsed.

16.8 Management

16.8.1 Acute pulmonary histoplasmosis

Few otherwise normal persons presenting with this form of histoplasmosis require treatment. In most cases spontaneous improvement has begun before the condition is diagnosed. Treatment is indicated in individuals whose symptoms are not improving after 2–3 weeks.

Patients with enlarged mediastinal lymph nodes sometimes require treatment to relieve symptoms of obstruction. Antifungal agents and corticosteroids can help to reduce lymph node enlargement, but neither have been beneficial in patients with mediastinal fibrosis. Surgical intervention to relieve obstruction has often proved difficult.

The traditional treatment of choice in patients who require active management is a short 2–4-week course of amphotericin B (0.5–0.7 mg/kg per day). Oral itraconazole (400 mg/day for 6 months) or ketoconazole (400 mg/day for at least 3 months) are also effective.

16.8.2 Chronic pulmonary histoplasmosis

If patients are seen in the initial stages of this illness and there is no cavitation and symptoms are mild, antifungal treatment can be withheld, provided signs of healing are observed. If symptoms progress or persist, antifungal treatment must be given. Surgical resection is no longer recommended.

Oral itraconazole (400 mg/day for 6 months) is the drug of choice for most patients with persistent cavitation. Oral ketoconazole (400 mg/day for 6–12 months) can also be used, but it is less well tolerated. Patients whose compliance with prolonged treatment is poor, and those requiring H2 antagonists or other drugs that impair itraconazole or ketoconazole absorption, should receive amphotericin B. The usual regimen is 0.5–0.7 mg/kg per day for 10 weeks. Patients should be followed-up for at least 12 months after treatment is discontinued.

16.8.3   Disseminated histoplasmosis

Treatment is essential for all patients with disseminated histoplasmosis, even those with a single focal lesion.

Oral itraconazole (400 mg/day) is the drug of choice for non-immunosuppressed patients with the milder, non-meningeal forms of chronic disseminated infection. However, amphotericin B remains the preferred treatment for patients with severe disseminated histoplasmosis. The usual regimen is 0.5–0.7 mg/kg per day for 10 weeks. Infants should receive 1.0 mg/kg for at least 6 weeks.

The management of patients with AIDS with disseminated histoplasmosis presents special problems. Treatment with amphotericin B (0.5–0.7 mg/kg per day) is often effective, but relapse is common when the drug is discontinued. Long-term maintenance treatment with a 1.0 mg/kg dose of amphotericin B at 1- or 2-week intervals has proved successful in some patients, but not in others.

Oral itraconazole is a safe and effective treatment for mild forms of disseminated histoplasmosis in patients with AIDS. The recommended dose is 400 mg/day for the first 12 weeks, and then 200 mg/day for long-term maintenance. Patients with AIDS with serious forms of disseminated histoplasmosis can be changed to itraconazole maintenance once their condition has improved on amphotericin B treatment. Maintenance treatment with fluconazole (400 mg/day) should be considered in patients with AIDS who fail to absorb itraconazole.

Oral ketoconazole is not recommended for induction or maintenance treatment of disseminated histoplasmosis in patients with AIDS.

17   Paracoccidioidomycosis

17.1   Definition

The term paracoccidioidomycosis is used to refer to infections due to the dimorphic fungus *Paracoccidioides brasiliensis*. Following inhalation this organism causes a benign and transient pulmonary infection in normal individuals. Later reactivation results in chronic infection of the lungs or other organs, in particular the skin and mucous membranes.

17.2   Geographical distribution

Most cases of paracoccidioidomycosis have been reported from South and Central America. However, the infection has also been diagnosed outside these regions among individuals who had earlier resided in or visited an endemic region.

17.3   The causal organism and its habitat

P. brasiliensis is a dimorphic fungus. It grows in nature as a mycelium, but in tissue it forms large oval or globose cells with characteristic multiple buds encircling the mother cell.

Although *P. brasiliensis* has been recovered from the soil on a few occasions, understanding of its natural habitat remains limited. In South and Central America, paracoccidioidomycosis is most frequently encountered in regions classified as subtropical mountain forests.

Skin testing of normal individuals living in endemic regions has demonstrated that infection with *P. brasiliensis* is often acquired before the age of 20 years. However, symptomatic paracoccidioidomycosis is most prevalent in individuals between the ages of 30 and 50 years. More than 90% of cases occur in men, most of whom have outdoor occupations. Epidemics of this mycosis have not been reported.

17.4   Clinical manifestations

Infection with *P. brasiliensis* follows inhalation of spores that have been released into the air. The lungs are the usual initial site of infection, but the organism then spreads through the lymphatics to the regional lymph nodes. Most normal individuals develop no symptoms or signs, but children and adolescents sometimes present with an acute disseminated form of infection in which superficial and/or visceral lymph node enlargement is the major manifestation.

Most patients with paracoccidioidomycosis present with chronic progressive infection which has resulted from reactivation of an old quiescent lesion. In some cases, the infection is confined to the lungs, but in others it has spread to involve the mucosa, skin or other organs. The disease is often indolent in onset, appearing long after an individual has left an endemic region. Most patients respond to anti-fungal treatment, but relapse is a common problem.

17.4.1 Chronic pulmonary paracoccidioidomycosis

In most cases this illness is insidious in onset and the patient has been ill for weeks or months before diagnosis. The most frequent symptoms include productive cough, fever, night sweats, malaise, haemoptysis and weight loss.

The radiological findings are characteristic, but not diagnostic. Multiple bilateral interstitial infiltrates are often found. If left untreated, these will progress to fibrosis and cavitation. Hilar lymph node enlargement is found in 50% of cases, but calcification and pleural effusion are uncommon. The lesions must be distinguished from histoplasmosis and tuberculosis.

17.4.2 Mucocutaneous paracoccidioidomycosis

Ulcerative mucocutaneous lesions are the most obvious presenting sign of chronic disseminated infection with *P. brasiliensis*.

The mouth and nose are the most common sites of mucosal infection. Painful ulcerated lesions develop on the gums, tongue, lips or palate and can progress over weeks or months, interfering with eating. Perforation of the palate or nasal septum may occur. Laryngeal lesions can lead to scar formation and ulceration resulting in hoarseness and stridor.

Cutaneous lesions often appear on the face around the mouth and nose, although patients with severe infection can have widespread scattered lesions. Small papular or nodular lesions enlarge over weeks or months into plaques with an elevated, well-defined margin. Verrucous lesions or ulcers with a rolled border may develop.

Lymphadenopathies are common in patients with buccal lesions. It is not uncommon for infection of the cervical lymph nodes to result in abscess formation and the development of draining sinuses.

17.4.3   **Other forms of disseminated paracoccidioidomycosis**
Haematogenous and lymphatic spread of *P. brasiliensis* can result in widespread disseminated infection. Manifestations include nodular or ulcerated lesions of the small or large intestine, hepatic and splenic lesions, adrenal gland destruction, osteomyelitis, arthritis, focal cerebral lesions and meningitis.

17.5   **Differential diagnosis**
Mucocutaneous leishmaniasis is endemic in the same regions as paracoccidioidomycosis and can cause similar lesions. The clinical and radiological manifestations of chronic *P. brasiliensis* infection of the lungs can be confused with tuberculosis or histoplasmosis.

17.6   **Essential investigations and their interpretation**
17.6.1   Microscopy
Microscopic examination of wet preparations of pus, sputum, crusts from granulomatous lesions and other clinical material can permit the diagnosis of paracoccidioidomycosis if the characteristic large round cells with multiple peripheral buds are seen. However, these are usually present as single cells or chains of cells and often cannot be differentiated from other fungal pathogens.

17.6.2   Culture
The definitive diagnosis of paracoccidioidomycosis depends on isolation of the fungus in culture. Mycelial colonies can be obtained after incubation at 25–30°C for 2–3 weeks, but cultures should be retained for 4 weeks before being discarded. Mycelial cultures seldom sporulate, but subculture of the isolate on blood agar at 37°C should result in production of the unicellular form. If more rapid identification is required (24 h), the initial mycelial culture can be subjected to an exoantigen test.

17.6.3   **Serological tests**

Serological tests are useful for the diagnosis of para-coccidioidomycosis. These tests have also been helpful for following the effect of treatment.

The complement fixation test is positive in more than 90% of patients with active paracoccidioidomycosis, higher titres being obtained in those with more severe infection. However, cross-reactions can occur with serum from patients with blastomycosis, histoplasmosis, sporotrichosis and several other infections.

The immunodiffusion test is positive in 80–90% of patients with active paracoccidioidomycosis. Although cross-reactions can occur in patients with histoplasmosis, these are uncommon.

Titres of antibodies decline on successful treatment, precipitins being the first to disappear. However, low titres may persist for a long time after cure of the infection.

17.7   **Management**

Patients with paracoccidioidomycosis require long-term antifungal treatment. Treated patients should be re-examined at regular intervals, because relapse is a common problem.

Oral itraconazole is the drug of choice for the treatment of paracoccidioidomycosis. The usual regimen is 100 mg/day given for 6 months. Late relapse has been uncommon, and relapsing patients have responded to further treatment with itraconazole. Oral ketoconazole is almost as effective, but less well tolerated than itraconazole. The usual dose is 200–400 mg/day given for up to 12 months (or for a minimum of 6 months after all clinical signs of infection have disappeared). If absorption of itraconazole or ketoconazole is a problem, oral or parenteral treatment with fluconazole (200–400 mg/day for 6 months) is also effective.

Amphotericin B remains a useful drug for the management of paracoccidioidomycosis. The usual regimen is 1.0 mg/kg per day for 4–8 weeks. Thereafter, treatment with a sulphonamide, such as sulphadiazine, should be administered for a further 6–12 months (or longer). The usual adult dose of sulphadiazine is 500–1000 mg at 4–6-h intervals. Children should receive 60–100 mg/kg per day in divided doses.

18   Chromoblastomycosis

18.1   Definition

The term chromoblastomycosis (chromomycosis) is used to refer to a chronic localized infection of the skin and subcutaneous tissue most often involving the limbs and characterized by raised crusted lesions. It may be caused by a number of brown-pigmented (dematiaceous) fungi.

18.2   Geographical distribution

The disease is most common in tropical and subtropical regions. Most cases occur in Central and South America, but chromoblastomycosis has also been reported in South Africa, Asia and Australia.

18.3   The causal organisms and their habitat

The disease is caused by various dematiaceous fungi, to which a number of names have been given. There is therefore a great deal of confusion in the nomenclature used by various authors.

The most common aetiological agents, in descending order, are *Phialophora verrucosa*, *Fonsecaea pedrosoi*, *Fonsecaea compacta*, *Cladophialophora* (*Cladosporium*) *carrionii* and *Rhinocladiella acquaspersa*. Sporadic cases of chromoblastomycosis have also been attributed to a number of other dematiaceous moulds. These organisms form characteristic thick-walled, dark-brown, muriform sclerotic cells in tissue.

The aetiological agents of chromoblastomycosis are widespread in the environment, being found in soil, wood and other plant materials. Infection follows the traumatic inoculation of the fungus into the skin and the disease is most prevalent among individuals with outdoor occupations and those who go barefoot. In most countries, chromoblastomycosis is more common in men than in women or children.

18.4   Clinical manifestations

Infection follows the traumatic introduction of the fungus

into the skin or subcutaneous tissue. Minor trauma, such as cuts or wounds due to thorns or wood splinters, is often sufficient to introduce the organism.

The clinical manifestations of chromoblastomycosis are similar, regardless of the organism causing it. The most common sites of infection are the lower legs and feet; other sites include the hands, arms, back and neck. In most cases, the lesions are unilateral.

The initial lesion is a small pink painless papule which develops at the site of implantation. However, most patients do not seek medical attention at this stage. If left untreated the initial lesion will increase in size and a large hyperkeratotic plaque, with a roughened surface and raised margin, will be formed. Lymphatic spread (and auto-inoculation) often results in the formation of satellite lesions around the original lesion. The condition is not painful, but itching often occurs. Even in cases where the disease has become widespread and involves an entire limb, the general health of the patient is not affected.

Later in the disease some lesions become pedunculated. Bacterial superinfection can occur, resulting in ulceration and a malodorous discharge. Superinfection is also thought to be responsible for the lymph stasis and elephantiasis that is seen in some patients with long-standing infection.

In occasional cases metastatic lesions develop in the lymph nodes, liver, brain or other tissues. As with other proliferative epidermal processes, the lesions can undergo carcinomatous transformation.

18.5 Differential diagnosis

Chromoblastomycosis must be distinguished from a number of other fungal infections including blastomycosis, lobomycosis, paracoccidioidomycosis, phaeohyphomycosis, rhinosporidiosis and sporotrichosis. It must also be differentiated from prototothecosis, leishmaniasis, cutaneous tuberculosis, certain leprous lesions, syphilis, psoriasis and subacute or discoid lupus erythematosus.

18.6 Essential investigations and their interpretation

18.6.1 Microscopy

Microscopic examination of tissue sections or wet preparations of pus, scrapings or biopsies from lesions can permit the diagnosis of chromoblastomycosis if clusters of the characteristic small, round, thick-walled, brown-pigmented sclerotic cells are seen. These cells are often divided by longitudinal and transverse septa.

18.6.2 Culture

The definitive diagnosis of chromoblastomycosis depends on the isolation of the aetiological agent in culture. Identifiable olive green–brownish black mycelial colonies can be obtained after incubation at 25–30°C for 1–2 weeks, but cultures should be retained for 4 weeks before being discarded. Identification of the individual aetiological agents is difficult.

18.7 Management

Chromoblastomycosis is a difficult condition to treat. Surgical excision should be reserved for small lesions. It carries a high risk of local dissemination and should only be attempted in conjunction with antifungal treatment.

There is no ideal medical treatment for chromoblastomycosis. However, long courses of oral itraconazole (200–600 mg/day for 12–36 months) have been reported to effect a marked improvement in a substantial proportion of South American patients with the infection.

Until the development of itraconazole, flucytosine (100–200 mg/kg per day given as four divided doses) was the drug of choice for chromoblastomycosis. However, resistance was a frequent problem. Much better results have been obtained when flucytosine is combined with amphotericin B (0.5–1.0 mg/kg per day) or oral thiabendazole (25 mg/kg per day). Treatment should be continued for at least 1 month after clinical cure is obtained.

The local application of heat to the lesions is sometimes beneficial.

19   Entomophthoramycoses

19.1   Rhinofacial conidiobolomycosis
19.1.1   Definition
This is a chronic localized subcutaneous fungal infection. It originates in the nasal mucosa and spreads to the adjacent subcutaneous tissue of the face causing severe disfigurement.

19.1.2   Geographical distribution
The disease is most common in West Africa, in particular Nigeria, but cases have also been reported from India and from South and Central America.

19.1.3   The causal organism and its habitat
Conidiobolus coronatus (*Entomophthora coronata*) is found in the soil and on decomposing vegetation in tropical rain forests. It is also an insect pathogen.

The disease is more common in men than in women or children. Most cases affect men living or working in tropical rain forests.

19.1.4   Clinical manifestations
Conidiobolus infection originates in the nasal mucosa, in the region of the inferior turbinates. In most cases the organism is introduced on the soiled hands of the patient himself. In some instances, the infection follows spore inhalation.

The most common symptom is nasal obstruction, which is often unilateral. Nasal discharge is a common finding, but pain, tenderness and constitutional upset are rare. The spread of the infection from the nose to the facial tissues is slow but relentless. Tissue swelling becomes pronounced, affecting the forehead, nose, cheeks and upper lip. It is this gross facial disfigurement that brings the patient for treatment.

The condition affects soft tissue, but the underlying bone is spared. The lesions have a distinct margin, but the mass is not movable over the underlying tissue. The skin is stretched, but remains intact.

19.1.5   **Differential diagnosis**

Even if, in advanced cases, the diagnosis is obvious from the typical clinical appearance, mycological and histological examinations are essential for its confirmation.

19.1.6   **Essential investigations and their interpretation**

MICROSCOPY

Microscopic examination of smears or tissue from the nasal mucosa will reveal characteristic, broad, non-septate, thin-walled mycelial filaments.

CULTURE

Cultures are far from simple to prepare, and the pathological material must be inoculated on the largest possible number of media; they should be incubated at between 25 and 35°C.

19.1.7   **Management**

Treatment of this condition is difficult, but patients often respond to oral itraconazole (200–400 mg/day) or ketoconazole (200–400 mg/day). Treatment should be continued for at least 1 month after the lesions have cleared.

Saturated potassium iodide solution is useful for patients in developing countries, because of its ease of administration and low cost. The starting dose is 1 ml three times daily, and this is increased up to 4–6 ml three times daily as tolerated. Treatment must be continued for at least 1 month after the lesions have disappeared. Allergic reactions and gastrointestinal intolerance are common complications, and relapse is common even long after successful treatment.

Surgical resection of infected tissue is seldom successful; it may hasten the spread of infection.

19.2   **Basidiobolomycosis**

19.2.1   **Definition**

This is a chronic subcutaneous fungal infection of the trunk and limbs.

19.2.2   **Geographical distribution**

The disease is most common in the tropical regions of East and West Africa, but cases have also been reported from India, the Middle East and Southeast Asia.

19.2.3   **The causal organism and its habitat**

Basidiobolus ranarum (*B. meristosporus*, *B. haptosporus*) has been isolated from decomposing vegetation lying on soil. It has also been recovered from the intestines of frogs, toads, lizards and other small reptiles.

Basidiobolomycosis is unusual among subcutaneous fungal infections in that it is more common in children and adolescents than in adults.

19.2.4   **Clinical manifestations**

It is still uncertain how the disease is acquired, but it is thought to follow traumatic inoculation. Minor trauma, such as a thorn prick or an insect bite, is often sufficient to introduce the organism.

The most common sites of infection are the buttocks and thighs, but the hard, movable subcutaneous swellings that characterize this condition are also found on the arms, legs or neck. Pain and tenderness are unusual. This is a disfiguring infection, but the skin covering the lesions remains intact. The underlying bone and joints are not affected. Lymphatic obstruction may occur and can result in elephantiasis.

19.2.5   **Differential diagnosis**

The clinical appearance of this disease is distinctive, but a firm diagnosis requires mycological and histological confirmation.

19.2.6   **Essential investigations and their interpretation**

MICROSCOPY

Microscopic examination of histopathological sections of infected tissue will reveal wide, irregular, non-septate filaments or fragments thereof.

CULTURE

Specimens should be cultured on glucose peptone agar at 30°C. Identifiable colonies should be obtained in less than 1 week.

19.2.7   **Management**

The therapy of choice still appears to be saturated potassium iodide solution (see section 19.1.7). In some cases co-trimoxazole has been found to be more effective than potassium iodide. The recommended dose is two tablets three times daily (each tablet contains 400 mg sulphamethoxazole and 80 mg trimethoprim). As with potassium iodide solution, treatment should be continued for 1 month after the lesions have cleared. Oral ketoconazole (400 mg/day) has sometimes been successful, but amphotericin B has seldom been helpful.

Should a patient have an enlarged, useless limb resistant to medical treatment, amputation should be considered, to forestall bacterial superinfection.

20   Lobomycosis

20.1   Definition
The term lobomycosis (keloidal blastomycosis) is used to refer to a rare, chronic infection of the skin and subcutaneous tissue due to the fungus *Loboa loboi*.

20.2   Geographical distribution
Most cases have come from the Amazon region of central Brazil and Surinam. Cases have also been reported from other countries in northern South America and Central America.

20.3   The causal organism and its habitat
The aetiological agent has been named *L. loboi*, but so far all attempts to isolate this fungus in culture have failed. In tissue it appears as round or elliptical budding cells. It is sometimes considered to be related to *Paracoccidioides brasiliensis*.

The natural habitat of *L. loboi* is still unknown. It is, however, accepted that it is a saprotroph in nature and that water has an important role in human infection. Lobomycosis has also been diagnosed in Atlantic dolphins, supporting the hypothesis of an aqueous habitat of the aetiological agent. Most human infections have occurred in individuals who resided in, or travelled through, the tropical rain forest regions of Central or South America. Most patients trace their infection to some traumatic incident, such as an insect bite, cut or abrasion. The disease is more common in men than in women or children. It is most prevalent in individuals between 30 and 40 years of age.

20.4   Clinical manifestations
The most common sites of infection are the legs and arms, face, ears and buttocks. The initial lesion is a papule or a small nodule which slowly proliferates to form extensive keloidal or verrucous lesions. The lesions are located in the dermis, the normal tissue being replaced by granulomatous tissue. Autoinoculation can lead to the development of

further lesions. In advanced cases, the lesions may cover an entire limb. In most instances the disease is symptomless. However, if the head is involved, the patient may be so grossly disfigured as to be completely excluded from social life.

20.5   Differential diagnosis

The vegetative lesions of lobomycosis must be distinguished from keloids, nodular lepromatous lesions, leishmaniasis and chromoblastomycosis.

20.6   Essential investigations and their interpretation

20.6.1   Microscopy

Histopathological examination of clinical material will reveal large numbers of the characteristic large round or oval thick-walled cells of *L. loboi* (over 10 μm in diameter). These can produce multiple buds that resemble the tissue form of *P. brasiliensis*. The cells are often formed in unbranched chains, the adjacent cells being joined together by bridge-like structures within the chain.

20.6.2   Culture

L. loboi has never been isolated in culture. This distinguishes it from *P. brasiliensis* to which it bears a marked resemblance.

20.7   Management

Antifungal treatment is ineffective, but oral clofazimine has given promising results in some patients. Provided the lesions are not too extensive, the treatment of choice is surgical excision. However, recurrence is common and patients should be followed up where possible.

21   Mycetoma

21.1   Definition

The term mycetoma is used to refer to a chronic localized destructive infection of the skin, subcutaneous tissue and bone. It usually affects the feet or hands and may be caused by various species of fungi (eumycetoma) or actinomycetes (actinomycetoma) which have been inoculated into subcutaneous tissue as a result of traumatic implantation. A characteristic feature of mycetoma is the production in infected tissue of grains which are compact masses of fungal or actinomycete elements, and their discharge to the outside through sinus tracts.

21.2   Geographical distribution

Mycetomas are most common in arid tropical and subtropical regions of Africa and Central and South America. The countries surrounding the Saharan and Arabian deserts form the most important endemic region, but the disease is also endemic in India and the Far East. Sporadic cases have been reported from other parts of the world.

21.3   The causal organisms and their habitat

More than 20 species of fungi and actinomycetes have been implicated as aetiological agents of mycetoma. Many of these organisms have been isolated from the soil or from living or decomposing vegetation. About six species of fungi are common causes of eumycetoma and five aerobic actinomycetes are common aetiological agents of actinomycetoma.

The predominant causes of mycetoma differ from one part of the world to another (see Table 21.1). In the arid regions of the tropics and subtropics, the most frequent aetiological agents are *Madurella mycetomatis*, *Actinomadura madurae*, *A. pelletieri* and *Streptomyces somaliensis*. In the humid mountain regions of Latin America, *Nocardia brasiliensis* is the predominant organism while *M. grisea* is a less prominent cause of infection. In temperate countries, the principal isolates have been *Scedosporium apiospermum*

Table 21.1 Aetiological agents of mycetoma.

Species	Geographical distribution	Colour of grain
Eumycetomas		
Leptosphaeria senegalensis	Africa	Black
Madurella grisea	Africa, Central and South America	Black
Madurella mycetomatis	Worldwide	Black
Neotestudina rosatii	Africa	White
Pyrenochaeta romeroi	Africa, South America	Black
Scedosporium apiospermum	Worldwide	White
Acremonium species	Africa, Middle East	White
Aspergillus nidulans	Africa, Middle East	White
Actinomycetomas		
Actinomadura madurae	Worldwide	White/yellow
Actinomadura pelletieri	Africa	Red
Nocardia asteroides	Worldwide	White/yellow
Nocardia brasiliensis	Central America	White/yellow
Streptomyces somaliensis	North Africa, Middle East	Yellow/brown

(*Pseudallescheria boydii*), *M. mycetomatis* and *Actinomadura madurae*. Other organisms that have sometimes been implicated as causes of mycetoma include *Leptosphaeria senegalensis*, *Neotestudina rosatii*, *Pyrenochaeta romeroi*, *Exophiala jeanselmei*, *Acremonium* species, *Aspergillus nidulans*, *N. asteroides* and *N. caviae*.

In some countries men are affected more frequently than women, but there is no consistent differential sex distribution. Mycetoma can affect all age groups, but is most common in individuals between 20 and 50 years of age. Most patients have outdoor occupations which expose them to soil and minor penetrating wounds.

21.4   Clinical manifestations

Infection follows the traumatic implantation of the pathogen into the skin or subcutaneous tissue. In some cases the organisms are introduced on thorns or wood splinters; in others infection is due to later contamination of the wound with soil organisms.

Mycetomas are most common on the feet (more than 70% of cases), particularly among those who go barefoot, followed by the hands (about 10% of cases) and other parts of the body that come into contact with the soil or vegetation during working, sitting or lying. Other frequently affected sites include the back, neck and back of the head, particularly in individuals who carry wood or loads contaminated with soil. In tropical countries patients most commonly present with long-standing infection.

The clinical features of the disease are similar, regardless of the organism causing it. The initial lesion, which appears several months after the traumatic incident, consists of a small firm painless subcutaneous nodule that can either be moved under the skin or is attached to it. In general, eumycetomas follow a slower and less destructive course than actinomycetomas. The former tend to remain localized and swelling and destruction of adjacent anatomical structures is not marked until late in the course of the disease. In actinomycetoma infections, the lesions have less well-defined margins and tend to merge with the surrounding tissue. Progression is often more rapid and involvement of bone earlier and more extensive.

Mycetoma lesions present as swellings covered with hypo- or hyperpigmented skin. The lesions develop single or multiple sinus tracts which discharge pus containing the characteristic grains onto the surface of the skin. As old sinus tracts heal, new ones appear. In time, the infection spreads to adjacent tissue, including bone. Depending on the location and size of the lesion, and also on any bone involvement, movement of the joints in the affected parts may be impaired. In spite of their unpleasant appearance, most mycetomas are painless, even when well established. However, in about 20% of cases pain is the main complaint that brings patients to hospital.

Radiological examination is useful in determining the extent of bone involvement. The most common and distinctive finding is focal bone destruction with formation of cavities. These are small and abundant in cases of actino-mycetoma and larger and less numerous in eumycetoma. Computed tomographic (CT) scans are also helpful in delineating the extent of the lesions.

Mycetomas often spread to adjacent tissues, but spread to the regional lymph nodes and involvement of deep organs is rare. Although lymphatic spread is found in some cases of eumycetoma, it is encountered more often in cases of acti-nomycetoma where the grains are smaller. In both cases repeated surgical interference seems to be an aggravating factor. Bacterial superinfection of the initial mycetoma lesion is common and is a frequent cause of regional lymph node enlargement and impairment of the general health of the patient.

21.5 Differential diagnosis

In most cases the diagnosis of mycetoma of the foot presents no problems, but it may be difficult if other body sites are involved, particularly if no grains have been discharged at the time of examination.

The characteristic feature of mycetoma is the presence in sinus tracts of grains which are found to contain actino-mycotic or fungal filaments. This finding distinguishes mycetoma from chromoblastomycosis, botryomycosis, cutaneous tuberculosis and other conditions.

21.6 Essential investigations and their interpretation

21.6.1 Gross examination

The diagnosis of mycetoma depends on the identification of grains. These should, if possible, be obtained by puncture from a softened, but not ulcerated, nodule with a syringe. Failing this, grains can be obtained with a dissecting needle or by aspiration from the secretion flowing from a sinus. If there is no pus flowing from the lesion, small fragments of tissue should be removed. If possible, 20–30 grains should be obtained; these should be rinsed in 70% alcohol, then washed in sterile saline before being cultured.

Gross examination of the grains may afford a clue as to the aetiological agent (see Table 21.1). Black grains suggest a fungal infection; minute white grains often indicate a *Nocardia* infection; larger white grains the size of a pinhead may be of either fungal or actinomycotic origin. Small red grains are specific to *Actinomadura pelletieri*, but yellowish-white grains may be actinomycotic or fungal in origin.

21.6.2 Microscopy

Direct microscopic examination will confirm the diagnosis of mycetoma, and will also reveal whether the causal organism is a fungus or an actinomycete. Actinomycotic grains contain very fine filaments (< 1 μm diameter) whereas fungal grains contain short hyphae (2–4 μm diameter) which are sometimes pigmented. This can be seen by direct microscopic examination of crushed grains in potassium hydroxide, but is much more readily observed in stained histological sections.

21.6.3 Culture

Although the identity of the causal agents of mycetoma can often be deduced from the morphological characteristics of the grains, it is also important to isolate the organism in culture. Agar plates should be inoculated with several grains (or with secretion or tissue fragments) and incubated at 25–30°C and at 37°C. The most commonly used agar medium is glucose peptone agar, without antibiotics but with cycloheximide (actidione) for isolation of actinomycetes, and with antibiotics but without cycloheximide for fungal agents. Alternative media for isolation of actinomycetes include brain–heart infusion or blood agar.

Cultures should be retained for up to 6 weeks before being discarded. The actinomycetes are much slower growing than the fungi.

21.7 Management

It is essential to distinguish eumycetomas from actinomycetomas because the treatment of these conditions is different, and the drugs used to treat one are ineffective in the other.

Medical treatment is often effective in cases of actinomycetoma. Good results have been obtained with streptomycin sulphate (1000 mg/day; intramuscular injection) given in combination with another drug. After the first month, the dosage interval can be increased to 48 h. Streptomycin treatment should be discontinued if ototoxic side-effects develop.

In cases of actinomycetoma due to *Actinomadura pelletieri* and *Nocardia brasiliensis*, and most cases due to *Streptomyces somaliensis*, streptomycin should be given in combination with co-trimoxazole (two tablets morning and evening; each tablet contains 400 mg sulphamethoxazole and 80 mg trimethoprim). In cases due to *A. madurae* and *S. somaliensis* which are resistant to co-trimoxazole, streptomycin should be combined with dapsone (200 mg/day). If no response is seen after 3 weeks of treatment, other drug regimens can be substituted. These include streptomycin plus rifampicin (600 mg/day) and streptomycin plus sulphadoxine-pyrimethamine (one Fansidar tablet twice per week; each tablet contains 500 mg sulphadoxine and 25 mg pyrimethamine).

In some cases, treatment of actinomycetoma results in anaemia and/or leucopenia. This is guarded against by prescribing iron and folic acid together with the specific treatment and assessing the full blood count at 2–3-week intervals.

The average duration of treatment of actinomycetoma is about 9 months. Treatment must be continued until the pain and swelling diminish, the discharge of secretion and grains stops, and the sinuses close. Even if these signs have disappeared, it is prudent to continue treatment for the same period of time as was required to achieve these results.

In most cases eumycetoma is unresponsive to antifungal treatment and radical surgical removal is the best option. Because eumycetoma infections are often localized and slow to spread, surgical excision is often successful, particularly if the lesions are small and there is no bone involvement. If bone is involved, amputation offers the only real hope of eradication. However, relapse is inevitable unless all traces of infection are removed. If the lesions affect the back, neck, back of the head, or other sites where excision or amputation is impossible, little can be done to help the patient.

There are several reports of successful treatment of eumycetoma due to *M. mycetomatis* and *Scedosporium apiospermum* with ketoconazole (400 mg/day for at least 9–12 months). Long-term treatment with itraconazole has resulted in improvement in *M. grisea* mycetoma. Medical management is justified in patients without bone disease and where regular supervision of the patient over a number of months is anticipated. Should the lesions fail to respond to antifungal treatment, surgical excision will be required.

22   Rhinosporidiosis

22.1   Definition

The term rhinosporidiosis is used to refer to an uncommon granulomatous infection of the nasal and other mucosa, due to *Rhinosporidium seeberi*.

22.2   Geographical distribution

The disease is most common in India and Sri Lanka, but sporadic cases have been reported from East Africa, Central America, Southeast Asia and other parts of the world.

22.3   The causal organism and its habitat

The aetiological agent is an endosporulating organism, *R. seeberi*. So far attempts to isolate this fungus in culture have failed. In tissue, *R. seeberi* forms abundant large thick-walled sporangia. Large numbers of spores are produced within the sporangia and, when mature, these are released through a pore in the wall. Each spore may develop to produce a new sporangium.

The mechanism by which human infection is acquired is not known, but it is believed that stagnant pools of fresh water are an important source. The disease is most prevalent in rural districts, among persons bathing in public ponds or working in stagnant water, such as rice fields. Rhinosporidiosis is most common in children and adolescents; males are more commonly affected than females.

22.4   Clinical manifestations

The nose is the most common site of rhinosporidiosis, being affected in more than 70% of cases. The fungus causes the production of large sessile or pedunculated lesions that affect one or both nostrils. The infection is insidious in onset and the patient remains unaware of its existence until symptoms of obstruction develop. Rhinoscopic examination will reveal papular or nodular, smooth-surfaced lesions that become pedunculated and acquire a papillomatous or proliferative appearance. The lesions are pink, red or purple in colour. If located low in the nostril, the polyps may protrude and hang onto the upper lip. In most cases the general health of the patient is unimpaired. Spontaneous remission is unusual and, left untreated, the polyps will continue to enlarge.

In some cases, lesions develop on the conjunctiva or the ears. Lesions may also appear on the penis and on the vulva or vagina in women. Cutaneous rhinosporidiosis is rare and is usually due to spread from a neighbouring mucosal lesion. It presents as minute papillomas which enlarge and become pedunculated. In most cases, skin lesions are asymptomatic.

22.5 Differential diagnosis

The appearance of pedunculated or unpedunculated polyps or nodules on the nasal mucosa or the conjunctiva should suggest the diagnosis of rhinosporidiosis. The presence of small white dots on the surface of the lesions is also helpful; on microscopic examination these are seen to be sporangia.

The condition must be distinguished from cryptococcosis, cutaneous tuberculosis, leprous lesions, leishmaniasis, and treponematoses. Lesions on the genitalia or anal region must be distinguished from warts, condylomata and haemorrhoids.

22.6 Essential investigations and their interpretation

22.6.1 Microscopy

Microscopic examination of tissue sections or wet preparations of tissue or discharge will reveal large round or oval sporangia up to 350 μm in diameter, with a thick wall and an operculum. The sporangia may be filled with endospores.

22.6.2 Culture

R. seeberi has never been isolated in culture.

22.7 Management

The treatment of choice is surgical excision of lesions, with or without cauterization. No drug treatment has proved effective. Recurrence is common and patients should be followed up where possible.

23 Sporotrichosis

23.1 Definition

The term sporotrichosis is used to refer to subacute or chronic infections due to the dimorphic fungus, *Sporothrix schenckii*. Following implantation this organism can cause cutaneous or subcutaneous infection which commonly shows lymphatic spread. Occasionally, infection of the lungs, joints, bones or other sites occurs in predisposed individuals.

23.2 Geographical distribution

Sporotrichosis is worldwide in distribution, but is most common in warm, temperate or tropical climatic regions. At present, the largest number of reported cases comes from the USA. Other regions where the infection is endemic include Central and South America, Africa and Australasia.

23.3 The causal organism and its habitat

The causative agent is a dimorphic fungus, *S. schenckii*, which is found in the soil, on plants, and on plant materials, such as wood and sphagnum moss. It grows in nature as a mycelium, but in tissue it forms small budding cells.

There is no clear sex, age or racial predilection, but sporotrichosis is more common in adults than children. The disease is most prevalent among individuals whose occupation brings them into contact with soil, plants or plant materials, such as gardeners, florists, mineworkers and carpenters. Most cases are sporadic, but epidemics sometimes occur in endemic regions. One of the largest outbreaks occurred in the South African gold mines in the 1940s when almost 3000 cases were recorded, the source of infection being contaminated timber used as pit props.

23.4 Clinical manifestations

Infection usually follows the traumatic implantation of *S. schenckii* into the skin or subcutaneous tissue. Minor trauma, such as abrasions or wounds due to thorns or wood splinters, is often sufficient to introduce the organism. In occasional cases, infection follows spore inhalation.

Sporotrichosis has a wide range of clinical manifestations. The most common presentation is a localized cutaneous or subcutaneous lesion. Lymphatic spread may then lead to the development of further cutaneous lesions. Much less commonly, the fungus may cause infection of the lungs, joints, bones and other sites. Widespread disseminated infection has been reported in diabetics, alcoholics, intravenous drug users and patients with the acquired immune deficiency syndrome (AIDS).

23.4.1 Cutaneous sporotrichosis

This is the most common clinical form of sporotrichosis. It tends to affect exposed sites, such as the limbs, and in particular the hands and fingers. The right hand is affected more frequently than the left.

The initial lesion, which usually appears 1–4 weeks after the traumatic incident, is a small firm painless nodule that is at first movable, but later becomes attached to the neighbouring tissue. The skin grows red, turns violaceous, and the nodule becomes soft and breaks down to form a persistent ulcer which discharges a serous or purulent fluid. The edge of the ulcer is often irregular and it may become oedematous and crusted.

Over the ensuing weeks and months, further nodules develop along the course of the lymphatics draining the site of the initial lesion. These in turn progress to ulceration. In about 25% of cutaneous infections, however, the initial lesion remains 'fixed' without lymphatic spread. Such infections are common in children and facial lesions also often behave in this manner.

In the disseminated cutaneous form of sporotrichosis, numerous papular or nodular lesions that progress to ulceration are distributed over the patient. This form of sporotrichosis is uncommon and it is usually seen in individuals with an underlying disease or predisposition. It is thought to follow lymphatic or haematogenous spread from an initial cutaneous or pulmonary focus of infection.

23.4.2 Extracutaneous sporotrichosis

Extracutaneous forms of sporotrichosis are most commonly seen in patients with an underlying disease or predisposition, such as diabetes mellitus, alcoholism or AIDS. The most common sites of involvement are the lungs, joints and bones, but occasional cases of endophthalmitis and meningitis have been reported.

Pulmonary sporotrichosis is an uncommon, chronic infection. It usually follows the inhalation of spores and is sometimes associated with enlargement of the hilar lymph nodes. In some cases, it follows haematogenous dissemination from another site of inoculation. The symptoms are non-specific and include productive cough, fever, weight loss, loss of appetite, breathlessness and haemoptysis. The latter can be massive and fatal. The most common radiological finding is upper lobe cavitation, similar to that seen in tuberculosis.

Arthritis results from the spread of an adjacent subcutaneous infection, or from direct inoculation into the joint, or from haematogenous dissemination. It is an indolent, progressive infection which tends to affect the knee and other large weight-bearing joints, although the small joints of the hand and wrist are sometimes involved. The most common symptoms are stiffness, pain and swelling of the affected joint.

In most cases, bone disease results from the spread of infection from an adjacent subcutaneous or joint lesion. In some cases, however, it occurs as a result of haematogenous dissemination. It is a chronic and indolent infection which tends to affect the long bones. Patients often complain of focal pain, with signs of focal tenderness and minimal swelling on examination. The most common radiological finding is a lytic lesion with a periosteal reaction. Most patients have concomitant arthritis.

Endophthalmitis, although rare, may result in blindness; chorioretinitis has also been reported. Occasional cases of meningitis have also been reported; the symptoms are identical to those of tuberculous meningitis.

23.5 Differential diagnosis

The development of a cutaneous lesion on the limbs following trauma is suggestive of sporotrichosis, at least if the patient is resident in an endemic region. The development of multiple ulcers along lymphatics is also suspicious.

Cutaneous forms of sporotrichosis must be distinguished from a wide range of infectious diseases, including blastomycosis, chromoblastomycosis, nocardiosis, paracoccidioidomycosis, leishmaniasis and cutaneous tuberculosis.

23.6 Essential investigations and their interpretation

23.6.1 Microscopy

Direct examination of clinical material, such as pus or tissue, is often disappointing because the organism is seldom abundant. However, the detection of typical oval or cigar-shaped cells or asteroid bodies of *S. schenckii* will confirm the diagnosis. Immunofluorescence staining is sometimes helpful in visualizing single fungal cells.

23.6.2 Culture

The definitive diagnosis of sporotrichosis depends on the isolation of the aetiological agent in culture. Clinical material should be inoculated onto several media, including glucose peptone agar, and incubated at 25–30°C. Identifiable mycelial colonies should appear in 3–5 days. The colour of the colonies usually changes from cream or light brown to dark brown or black with age. Confirmation of the identification depends on the morphological characteristics of the mycelial form and its conversion to the yeast form on blood agar at 37°C.

23.6.3 Serological tests

At present, serological tests do not have a significant role in the diagnosis of sporotrichosis. Immunodiffusion and agglutination tests can be used to detect antibodies to *S. schenckii*, but are more helpful in diagnosing the unusual extracutaneous forms of sporotrichosis than in detecting cutaneous infection.

23.7 Management

Oral itraconazole is the drug of choice for patients with cutaneous and lymphocutaneous forms of sporotrichosis. It should be given at a dosage of 100–200 mg/day for 3–6 months. Treatment should be continued for several months after the lesions have cleared. Fluconazole is less effective, and should be regarded as a second-line treatment for patients who do not tolerate or cannot absorb itraconazole. The minimum dosage should be 400 mg/day. Oral ketoconazole is usually ineffective in lymphocutaneous sporotrichosis.

Saturated potassium iodide solution remains a useful treatment for patients in developing countries who contract lymphocutaneous sporotrichosis, because of its ease of administration and low cost. The starting dose is 1 ml three times daily, and this is increased to 4–6 ml three times daily. Treatment should be continued for at least a month after clinical cure is obtained, which may take 2–4 months. Allergic reactions and gastrointestinal intolerance are common complications of potassium iodide treatment.

The less common extracutaneous forms of sporotrichosis are difficult to treat. Potassium iodide is ineffective in osteoarticular sporotrichosis. Amphotericin B has cured some patients, but better results have been obtained when medical treatment has been combined with surgical debridement.

Itraconazole (400 mg/day) is the treatment of choice for patients with osteoarticular forms of sporotrichosis. Treatment should be continued for at least 12 months; shorter courses have led to relapse. Fluconazole (400–800 mg/day) is less effective, and should be reserved for the occasional patient who cannot be treated with itraconazole.

The treatment of pulmonary sporotrichosis is difficult and relapse is a common problem. Patients who are acutely ill should be treated with amphotericin B (1.0 mg/kg per day), but itraconazole (400 mg/day) may be substituted once their condition has improved. Patients who are not severely ill may be treated with itraconazole from the outset. Many patients with pulmonary sporotrichosis have underlying chronic obstructive pulmonary disease that precludes surgical resection of lesions.

Patients with life-threatening disseminated sporotrichosis require amphotericin B treatment (1.0 mg/kg per day). This should be continued until a total dose of 1–2 g has been administered. Patients with less acute forms of disseminated infection may be treated with itraconazole (400 mg/day) from the outset. Patients with AIDS with sporotrichosis require life-long maintenance treatment with itraconazole to prevent relapse.

Local application of heat is an effective alternative treatment for cutaneous or lymphocutaneous sporotrichosis in patients who are intolerant of the drugs used in these infections.

24   Hyalohyphomycosis

24.1   Definition

The term hyalohyphomycosis is used to refer to infections due to colourless (hyaline) moulds that adopt a septate hyphal form in tissue. This all-encompassing term was introduced in an attempt to stem the proliferation of new disease names each time an organism belonging to a new fungal genus was incriminated as the cause of infection. The number of organisms identified as causal agents of hyalo-hyphomycosis is increasing with over 40 different organisms, classified in 23 genera, being listed to date. The term hyalohyphomycosis is reserved as a general name for infections that are caused by unusual hyaline moulds that are not the cause of otherwise-named infections, such as aspergillosis.

24.2   *Fusarium* infection

24.2.1   Geographical distribution

These infections are worldwide in distribution. However, most cases of disseminated *Fusarium* infection have been reported from North America or from Mediterranean countries.

24.2.2   The causal organisms and their habitat

Members of the genus *Fusarium* are common soil organisms and important plant pathogens. The most frequent cause of human infection is *F. solani*, but *F. oxysporum*, *F. moniliforme* and at least 12 other species have also been implicated. The identification of these moulds is difficult and often confusing, even for specialists, and it is not surprising that the species of *Fusarium* involved has not been determined in over 50% of published reports.

24.2.3   Clinical manifestations

Fusarium species have long been recognized as one of the most frequent causes of corneal infection (see Chapter 8). Localized deep tissue infection is rarer, but cases of endophthalmitis, osteomyelitis and arthritis have been reported following the traumatic introduction of the organism. Occasional cases of paranasal sinus infection have been described.

Disseminated *Fusarium* infection is most commonly encountered in neutropenic cancer patients and bone marrow transplant (BMT) recipients, but cases have also been reported in burns patients and other debilitated or immunocompromised individuals. Many of these infections follow inhalation, but some have originated from cutaneous lesions associated with infected nails.

The clinical manifestations of disseminated *Fusarium* infection are similar in several respects to those of aspergillosis (see Chapter 10). Like the aetiological agents of aspergillosis and mucormycosis, *Fusarium* species have a predilection for vascular invasion, resulting in thrombosis and tissue necrosis. The most common presentation in the neutropenic patient is a persistent fever (greater than 38°C) that is unresponsive to broad-spectrum antibacterial treatment.

Identical cutaneous lesions occur in both *Aspergillus* and *Fusarium* infection, but are much more common in the latter. Three forms of cutaneous or subcutaneous lesion have been described: (i) painful, erythematous, macules or papules that evolve into black necrotic ulcers, similar to the ecthyma-gangrenosum-like lesions seen in patients with aspergillosis (see Chapter 10); (ii) target lesions which consist of ecthyma-gangrenosum-like lesions with an additional thin erythematous margin; and (iii) multiple erythematous subcutaneous nodules. In addition, extensive cellulitis of the face or limbs, with or without fasciitis can also occur. Cutaneous lesions occur in about 70% of patients with *Fusarium* infection, compared with less than 5% of patients with aspergillosis.

24.2.4   **Essential investigations and their interpretation**

The diagnosis of *Fusarium* infection depends on the isolation of the aetiological agent in culture because the hyphal tissue form of these moulds cannot be distinguished from that of other agents of hyalohyphomycosis or aspergillosis on microscopic examination. Infection with *Fusarium* has been associated with a much higher rate of isolation from blood culture (about 60% of cases) than has been the case with *Aspergillus* and other mould infections. However, it has not been established whether lysis-centrifugation is any more useful than other blood culture systems. *Fusarium* can usually be isolated from biopsies of cutaneous lesions.

24.2.5 Management

The most important factors influencing the outcome of *Fusarium* infection are the underlying condition of the patient and the extent of the infection.

Most patients who have developed disseminated *Fusarium* infection have been neutropenic and many have died before the disease is suspected. Even with high-dose amphotericin B treatment (1.0–1.5 mg/kg per day), the prognosis is poor unless the neutrophil count recovers. There are numerous regimens for administration of this drug, but widespread agreement that in immunocompromised patients it is essential to give the full dose from the outset (see Chapter 3). Limited clinical experience suggests that shortening the duration of neutropenia with colony-stimulating factors may be beneficial in treating disseminated *Fusarium* infection.

Administration of one of the lipid-based forms of amphotericin B should be considered in patients who fail to respond to the conventional formulation, or who develop side-effects that necessitate discontinuation of the drug, or in whom the conventional formulation is contraindicated because of renal impairment. There are different dosage recommendations for the various lipid-based preparations (see Chapter 3). It remains unclear as to whether these new formulations differ from each other or the conventional form in terms of clinical benefit in *Fusarium* infection.

Non-immunosuppressed individuals with localized *Fusarium* infection of soft tissue or bone often respond to treatment. Amphotericin B (1.0 mg/kg per day) remains the agent of choice for patients with osteomyelitis, but successful management often requires aggressive surgical debridement of necrotic tissue. Patients with endophthalmitis require both medical and surgical treatment. Intravitreal concentrations of amphotericin B following parenteral administration are too low to treat this infection and intravitreal instillation is required. This will result in inflammation and retinal damage, but doses up to 10 µg can be tolerated. Surgical debridement is an essential part of the management of this infection.

Itraconazole and fluconazole have been used in too few patients with *Fusarium* infection for their usefulness to be assessed. Both agents appear to be ineffective in tests *in vitro*, but correlation of MICs with clinical outcome have not been established.

24.3 *Scedosporium* infection

24.3.1 Geographical distribution

These infections are worldwide in distribution.

24.3.2 The causal organisms and their habitat

Two members of the genus *Scedosporium* have been implicated as aetiological agents of human infection. *Scedosporium apiospermum* (the current name for the imperfect form of the ascomycete *Pseudallescheria boydii*) is a ubiquitous, soil-inhabiting fungus. Infection can follow traumatic implantation, inhalation or aspiration of contaminated water. *S. prolificans* (which used to be named *S. inflatum*) is a rarer cause of human infection, but one which appears to be resistant to all available antifungal agents. The natural habitat of *S. prolificans* has not been identified, but it is thought to be a soil inhabitant.

24.3.3 Clinical manifestations

S. apiospermum and *S. prolificans* have emerged as significant causes of fungal infection in both normal and immunocompromised individuals. Localized soft-tissue and bone infections have occurred in non-compromised persons following traumatic inoculation. In immunocompromised patients inhalation of spores has resulted in fatal disseminated infection.

S. apiospermum is the most frequent cause of fungal mycetoma in temperate regions. This chronic infection results from the traumatic implantation of the fungus into subcutaneous tissue (see Chapter 21). The feet and hands are the most common sites of infection. The initial lesion, which appears several months after the traumatic incident, is a small painless subcutaneous nodule. This enlarges and ruptures to the surface forming sinus tracts which discharge white grains, then spreads into adjacent tissue and bone, causing disfiguring swelling and tissue destruction.

The lung is the second most common site of *Scedospor-*

ium infection in humans. In the immunocompetent individual, isolation of these moulds from sputum most commonly represents transient (or more prolonged)
colonization of the bronchi or lungs or both. Underlying
cavitating or cystic lung disease is a major factor predisposing an individual to *Scedosporium* colonization. Fungus
ball formation has been described in patients with residual
tuberculous or bronchiectatic cavities.

Scedosporium pneumonia is rare in immunocompetent
individuals. However, it has been seen following the
aspiration of contaminated water. Fatal dissemination to
the brain is a frequent complication.

In immunosuppressed patients, the clinical manifestations
of *Scedosporium* infection of the lungs are similar to those of
invasive aspergillosis (see Chapter 10). The most common
presentation in the neutropenic patient is a persistent fever
(greater than 38°C) that is unresponsive to broad-spectrum
antibacterial treatment. Many have developed a disseminated infection.

Localized deep forms of *Scedosporium* infection can
follow traumatic introduction of the fungus into soft tissue or
its dissemination from the lungs. Osteomyelitis, arthritis,
sinusitis, endophthalmitis, endocarditis, meningitis and focal
brain lesions have been reported in non-immunosuppressed
individuals. Corneal infection has also been described.

24.3.4 Essential investigations and their interpretation

The diagnosis of *Scedosporium* infection rests on the isolation of the fungus from clinical specimens because the
hyphal tissue form of these moulds cannot be distinguished
from that of other aetiological agents of hyalohyphomycosis
or aspergillosis in wet preparations or sections. This distinction is important because the different moulds in these
infections differ in their response to antifungal agents.

The organisms have been isolated from cerebrospinal
fluid (CSF) specimens in patients with meningitis, but blood
cultures are seldom positive.

24.3.5 Management

Surgical resection remains the preferred treatment for
patients with localized cavitating lesions of the lung. Other
localized forms of *Scedosporium* infection, such as sinusitis,

arthritis and osteomyelitis, have also been eradicated following surgical debridement of infected tissue. In some cases cure has resulted when debridement has been combined with antifungal treatment.

Many strains of *S. apiospermum* are resistant to amphotericin B and infections with this mould are best treated with an azole, such as parenteral miconazole, or oral ketoconazole (400–600 mg/day). Itraconazole (400 mg/day) has also proved effective in some patients.

S. prolificans appears to be resistant to all currently available antifungal agents and the prognosis for immuno-compromised patients with disseminated infection is dismal.

24.4 Other agents of hyalohyphomycosis

Many other colourless moulds have been incriminated as occasional aetiological agents of human hyalohyphomycosis. Isolation of these organisms alone is insufficient grounds for making a diagnosis because many are common culture contaminants. Even when the same organism is recovered on more than one occasion, the diagnosis must remain in doubt unless the fungus is demonstrated in histopathological sections.

Paecilomyces lilacinus is a common culture contaminant and its isolation must be interpreted with caution. However, this mould has caused outbreaks of endophthalmitis in surgical patients following its inadvertent administration in contaminated irrigation fluids. Fatal endocarditis has followed heart valve replacement and sinusitis has also been reported.

Scopulariopsis brevicaulis, a mould more commonly associated with onychomycosis (see Chapter 7), has caused fatal disseminated infection in neutropenic patients. As in patients with *Fusarium* infection, cutaneous lesions adjacent to infected toenails have been identified as the source of a subsequent disseminated infection.

25 *Penicillium marneffei* infection

25.1 Definition

Penicillium marneffei infection has become one of the most frequent opportunistic infections encountered in patients with the acquired immune deficiency syndrome (AIDS) who have resided in or visited Southeast Asia or southern China. This disease can also occur in normal individuals. Infection is thought to follow inhalation, but widespread disseminated infection is the most common clinical presentation.

25.2 Geographical distribution

Most cases of *P. marneffei* infection have been reported from Southeast Asia, in particular northern Thailand, and southern China. However, the infection has also been diagnosed outside this region among individuals who had earlier resided in or visited an endemic region.

25.3 The causal organism and its habitat

P. marneffei is a dimorphic fungus. It exists in nature as a mycelium, but in tissue it forms small round to elliptical cells which divide by fission.

Thus far, the natural habitat of *P. marneffei* has not been identified, but the soil appears to be an important reservoir for human infection. The fungus has been isolated from four different species of bamboo rats in Southeast Asia, but the relationship to human illness is uncertain.

Until the late 1980s few natural human infections with *P. marneffei* had been reported, and these had all occurred in individuals living in Southeast Asia or visiting the region. However, following the spread of AIDS to this region, *P. marneffei* infection has become much more common. It is now the third most common opportunistic infection among patients with AIDS living in northern Thailand. In addition, numerous cases of *P. marneffei* infection have been diagnosed in European and North American patients with AIDS who had become infected during visits to Southeast Asia.

P. marneffei infection is more common in the north of

Thailand, where up to 25% of patients with AIDS are affected, than in the south and Bangkok, where no more than 2% are infected. There is evidence of seasonal variation in the incidence of infection, with the highest incidence occurring during the rainy season from May to October. Most European and North American patients with AIDS with *P. marneffei* infection have only spent short periods of time in Southeast Asia and few have visited the recognized endemic regions. This suggests that the organism may be more widespread than has been suspected. It also suggests that patients with AIDS can acquire the infection following the minimum of exposure.

25.4   Clinical manifestations

Infection with *P. marneffei* is thought to follow inhalation of spores that have been released into the air. The lungs are the usual initial site of infection, but most affected individuals present with widespread disseminated infection. In some cases this results from the late reactivation of an old quiescent lesion during immunosuppression. In others, active infection occurs within a few weeks of exposure in an endemic region.

Patients with *P. marneffei* infection often present with a chronic progressive illness. The most common symptoms include fever, marked weight loss and debilitation. Many patients present with multiple papular skin lesions, some of which show central necrotic umbilication, resembling molluscum contagiosum. Other presenting signs include generalized lymphadenitis, hepatosplenic enlargement, anaemia and thrombocytopenia. Some patients have osteolytic bone lesions or subcutaneous abscesses. The illness is usually fatal if left untreated.

Chest radiographs often reveal diffuse reticulonodular or localized alveolar infiltrates. Pleural effusion and hilar lymph node calcification are uncommon.

25.5   Differential diagnosis

Histoplasmosis and cryptococcosis are endemic in the same regions as *P. marneffei* infection and can cause similar necrotic skin lesions in patients with AIDS. The radiological signs of *P. marneffei* infection can be confused with those of pulmonary tuberculosis.

25.6   **Essential investigations and their interpretation**

It is recommended that patients with AIDS who have visited Southeast Asia should be investigated for signs of *P. marneffei* infection if they present with fever, cutaneous lesions, lung disease, generalized lymphadenitis, or hepatosplenic enlargement.

25.6.1   Microscopy

Microscopic examination of Wright-stained bone marrow smears or touch smears of skin or lymph node biopsies can permit the diagnosis of *P. marneffei* infection if the characteristic round, oval or elliptical cells, often with prominent cross-walls are seen (often within macrophages). *P. marneffei* cells can, however, be confused with those of *Histoplasma capsulatum*. However, unlike the latter, *P. marneffei* cells often possess cross-walls, but never produce buds.

25.6.2   Culture

The definitive diagnosis of *P. marneffei* infection depends on isolation of the fungus in culture. The organism has been isolated from skin and lymph node biopsies, pus, bone marrow aspirates, sputum, bronchoalveolar lavage fluid and other clinical materials. It has been recovered from blood cultures in over 70% of cases in patients with AIDS.

Identifiable mycelial colonies can be obtained on glucose peptone agar after incubation at 25–30°C for 1 week, but cultures should be retained for up to 3 weeks before being discarded. *P. marneffei* colonies produce a distinctive red pigment which diffuses into the agar. However, some other non-pathogenic species of *Penicillium* can also produce a similar pigment.

25.7   **Management**

P. marneffei infection is a treatable condition, but delay may be fatal.

Amphotericin B remains the drug of choice for patients with severe *P. marneffei* infection. The usual regimen is 1.0 mg/kg per day for 2 weeks. Patients can then be changed to itraconazole (200–400 mg/day) or ketoconazole (400 mg/day) for a further 6 weeks, provided their condition has improved on amphotericin B treatment. In milder infections, itraconazole or ketoconazole can be used from the outset.

Fluconazole appears to be less effective than itraconazole, but it may be useful in patients who fail to absorb the latter drug.

Long-term maintenance treatment with oral itraconazole (200 mg/day) is recommended for patients with AIDS with *P. marneffei* infection, because relapse is common when antifungals are discontinued.

26   Phaeohyphomycosis

26.1   **Definition**

The term phaeohyphomycosis is used to refer to sub-cutaneous and deep-seated infections due to brown-pigmented (dematiaceous) moulds that adopt a septate mycelial form in tissue. This term was introduced in an attempt to stem the proliferation of new disease names each time an organism belonging to a new fungal genus was identified as the cause of human infection. This term was also created to segregate various clinical infections due to dematiaceous moulds from the distinctive subcutaneous infection known as chromoblastomycosis (see Chapter 18).

26.2   **Geographical distribution**

Phaeohyphomycosis has a worldwide distribution, but subcutaneous infection is most often seen in the rural population of tropical parts of Central and South America. Most cases of cerebral or paranasal sinus infection have been reported from North America.

26.3   **The causal organisms and their habitat**

The number of organisms implicated as aetiological agents of phaeohyphomycosis is increasing. More than 100 different moulds, classified in 60 different genera, have been incriminated. Often these fungi have been given different names at different times and there is therefore a great deal of confusion in the nomenclature used in different reports.

Among the more important aetiological agents can be included *Alternaria* species, *Bipolaris* species, *Cladophialophora* (*Xylohypha*) *bantiana*, *Curvularia* species, *Exophiala* species, *Exserohilum* species and *Phialophora* species. Many of these organisms are found in the soil or decomposing plant materials; others are plant pathogens. Human infection follows inhalation or traumatic implantation of the fungus.

One common factor among these fungi is their melanin formation in the cell wall in culture and, in most cases, in human tissue.

26.4   **Clinical manifestations**

Phaeohyphomycosis can be divided into a number of distinct clinical forms, including subcutaneous infection, paranasal sinus infection and cerebral infection.

26.4.1   **Subcutaneous phaeohyphomycosis**

This form of phaeohyphomycosis usually follows the traumatic implantation of the fungus into the subcutaneous tissue. Minor trauma, such as cuts or wounds due to thorns or wood splinters is often sufficient to introduce the organism. The principal aetiological agents include *Exophiala jeanselmei*, *E. spinifera*, *E. dermatitidis* (*Wangiella dermatitidis*), *Phialophora richardsiae* and *P. parasitica.*

The clinical manifestations of subcutaneous phaeohyphomycosis are similar regardless of the organism causing it. The most common sites of infection are the arms and legs; other sites include the buttocks, neck and face.

The initial lesion is a firm, sometimes tender, subcutaneous nodule. If left untreated this will slowly increase in size to form a painless cystic abscess. In most cases the lesions remain localized; the overlying skin usually remains unaffected. Purulent fluid can be aspirated from well-developed abscesses.

Draining sinuses sometimes develop in immunocompromised patients with subcutaneous phaeohyphomycosis.

26.4.2   **Paranasal sinus infection**

This form of phaeohyphomycosis is becoming more common. It occurs in both immunocompetent and immunosuppressed individuals. The principal aetiological agents include *Alternaria* species, *Bipolaris spicifera*, *B. hawaiiensis*, *Curvularia lunata* and *Exserohilum rostratum.*

Phaeohyphomycotic sinusitis is a slowly progressive, destructive condition that may remain confined to the sinuses or spread to the orbit and brain. The clinical presentation is similar to that of *Aspergillus* sinusitis (see Chapter 10). Affected individuals usually complain of long-standing symptoms of allergic rhinitis, nasal polyps, or intermittent sinus pain. Patients present with nasal obstruction and facial pain, with or without proptosis. The sinuses are filled with a thick dark inspissated mucus. Computed tomographic (CT) scans can be used to determine the extent of the infection.

Several dematiaceous moulds have been reported to cause black necrotic lesions on the nasal mucosa in patients with leukaemia or the acquired immune deficiency syndrome (AIDS). These lesions are identical to those seen in immunocompromised patients with aspergillosis (see Chapter 10).

26.4.3 Cerebral phaeohyphomycosis

This uncommon, but often lethal form of phaeohyphomycosis may follow haematogenous dissemination of infection from the lungs or it may result from direct spread from the nasal sinuses. Most cases are due to *Cladophialophora* (*Xylohypha*) *bantiana*. Other aetiological agents include *Bipolaris* species and *Exophiala* (*Wangiella*) *dermatitidis*. Many cases of *C. bantiana* brain abscess have occurred in immunocompetent individuals with no obvious risk factors predisposing them to this infection. More cases have been reported in men than women.

The symptoms of cerebral phaeohyphomycosis are gradual in onset. Persistent headache is the most common presenting symptom. The most frequent clinical findings include focal neurological signs, hemiparesis and fits. Fever is minimal or absent. Chest radiographs are normal.

CT scans are helpful in locating the lesions. Scans will often reveal a well-circumscribed lesion with a contrast-enhancing margin. The frontal lobes of the brain are the most common location. The cerebrospinal fluid (CSF) findings are varied. The opening pressure may be raised, the protein concentration may be increased, the glucose concentration may be reduced, and pleocytosis may be present. It is most unusual to recover the fungus from the CSF.

The diagnosis is seldom established until the lesion is resected.

26.4.4 Cutaneous infection

Several dematiaceous moulds (including *Alternaria* species) have been seen in, and isolated from, crusted, ulcerated or scaling skin lesions. Many of these infections have followed traumatic implantation and a substantial proportion have occurred in neutropenic patients or transplant recipients. The arms and legs are the most common sites of infection.

26.4.5 Other forms of phaeohyphomycosis

Several dematiaceous moulds have caused endocarditis

following valve insertion or replacement and peritonitis in patients on continuous peritoneal dialysis. Post-traumatic osteomyelitis and arthritis have also been reported.

26.5 Differential diagnosis

The lesions of subcutaneous phaeohyphomycosis can be confused with the small initial lesions of chromoblastomycosis, sporotrichosis, blastomycosis, coccidioidomycosis and paracoccidioidomycosis, as well as with cutaneous leishmaniasis. Lymphangitic spread of sporotrichosis and the development of verrucous lesions in the other conditions makes the distinction easier.

In immunocompetent individuals, the clinical presentation of phaeohyphomycotic sinusitis is indistinguishable from that of *Aspergillus* infection (see Chapter 10). In immunosuppressed patients, *Aspergillus* sinusitis is a fulminant, often lethal, condition unlike phaeohyphomycosis. However, both groups of organisms have caused black necrotic lesions of the nasal septum in patients with leukaemia or AIDS.

The presenting symptoms of cerebral phaeohyphomycosis are similar to those of an untreated bacterial brain abscess, but the fungal infection is often more indolent in onset. In occasional patients, the diagnosis of cryptococcosis, histoplasmosis, coccidioidomycosis or sporotrichosis must be excluded.

26.6 Essential investigations and their interpretation

26.6.1 Microscopy

Microscopic examination of stained tissue sections or wet preparations of clinical material, such as pus, scrapings or biopsies from lesions can permit the diagnosis of phaeohyphomycosis if brown-pigmented septate mycelium with occasional branching is seen.

26.6.2 Culture

Identification of the aetiological agent is often essential for correct management and this depends on its isolation in culture. Identifiable mycelial colonies can be obtained after incubation at 30°C for 1–3 weeks.

26.7	**Management**
26.7.1	Subcutaneous phaeohyphomycosis

Incision and drainage of subcutaneous lesions is seldom successful. Surgical resection is required. Treatment with amphotericin B has cured or improved non-resectable lesions, but later relapse has been common.

26.7.2	Paranasal sinus infection

Complete surgical resection of lesions combined with amphotericin B treatment is essential to halt the progression of phaeohyphomycotic sinusitis. Even so, it is not uncommon for the condition to recur, necessitating further surgical intervention. The need for repeated debridement is most evident in patients with disabling symptoms or erosion of the bone separating the paranasal sinus from the brain.

Oral treatment with itraconazole (100–400 mg/day) appears promising, although the optimum dosage and duration of treatment has not been defined.

Necrotic nasal septum lesions have been cured following surgical excision.

26.7.3	Cerebral phaeohyphomycosis

This infection requires both surgical and medical treatment: amphotericin B on its own is ineffective. Surgical resection of solitary lesions has resulted in some long-term cures. However, lesions that have not been completely removed have usually proved fatal. Patients with multifocal lesions have a poor prognosis.

26.7.4	Cutaneous infection

Surgical debridement of cutaneous lesions combined with parenteral amphotericin B is the most effective form of management. Topical antifungal treatment is seldom helpful.

26.7.5	Other forms of phaeohyphomycosis

Too few patients have been treated to make firm recommendations. However, the response to amphotericin B has been partial at best. Surgical resection of lesions or oral treatment with itraconazole should be considered.

27   Uncommon yeast infections

27.1   Introduction

In recent years a number of yeast species that had previously been thought to represent contamination or harmless colonization when isolated from humans have been recognized as significant pathogens in compromised patients. Establishing the diagnosis is difficult and depends on the detection of the organism in tissue sections or smears of clinical material as well as isolation in culture.

27.2   Trichosporonosis

In addition to causing white piedra, an uncommon asymptomatic infection of the scalp, facial and pubic hair (see Chapter 6), *Trichosporon beigelii* (which used to be named *T. cutaneum*) can also cause a deep-seated infection known as trichosporonosis in immunocompromised individuals. A second species, *T. capitatum* (which has now been reclassified as *Blastoschizomyces capitatus*) has been implicated as the cause of similar infections.

27.2.1   Geographical distribution

These infections are worldwide in distribution.

27.2.2   The causal organisms and their habitat

Trichosporon species have a widespread natural distribution, being found in soil and water and on plants. They are also carried on the mucosal and cutaneous surfaces of humans. Most cases of trichosporonosis appear to be derived from an endogenous reservoir of organisms in the gastrointestinal tract.

27.2.3   Clinical manifestations

Localized deep infection with *T. beigelii* has been reported in individuals with a serious underlying medical condition or other major predisposing factors. *T. beigelii* has caused endophthalmitis, endocarditis and peritonitis in individuals with disrupted anatomical barriers. The clinical presentation is similar to candidosis (see Chapter 11). *Trichosporon* infection of the lungs has been reported in leukaemic patients, most of whom had normal neutrophil counts.

Disseminated trichosporonosis is an uncommon but often lethal infection in immunosuppressed individuals. Most cases have occurred in neutropenic cancer patients and bone marrow transplant (BMT) recipients, but the infection has also been seen in solid organ transplant recipients and patients with the acquired immune deficiency syndrome (AIDS). Over 100 cases of disseminated infection with *T. beigelii* have been reported, most of which have had a fatal outcome.

The clinical manifestations of disseminated trichosporonosis are similar in most respects to those of disseminated candidosis (see Chapter 11). Like candidosis, trichosporonosis may take the form of an acute or a chronic infection. The former often presents as a persistent fever that fails to respond to broad-spectrum antibacterial treatment. Necrotic cutaneous lesions are often found. The liver, spleen, lungs and gastrointestinal tract are among the organs which may be involved. Chronic disseminated infection often begins while the patient is neutropenic, but does not become apparent until after the neutrophil count has recovered. The patient remains febrile and unwell, developing an enlarged liver and spleen.

27.2.4 Essential investigations and their interpretation

The diagnosis of trichosporonosis is seldom suspected until the fungus is isolated from blood, urine or cutaneous lesions. Often, however, patients have died and the infection has remained unrecognized until material obtained post-mortem has been investigated.

MICROSCOPY

Microscopic examination of smears and histopathological sections of cutaneous lesions will reveal branching hyphae with numerous rectangular arthrospores and budding blastospores. If arthrospores are sparse in tissue, *T. beigelii* can resemble *Candida albicans*. However, *T. beigelii* sometimes produces more true hyphae and fewer pseudohyphae than *C. albicans*.

CULTURE

In culture, members of the genus *Trichosporon* form white

to cream, heaped colonies that consist of hyaline mycelium with arthrospores and blastospores. In neutropenic patients, blood cultures are often positive and the organisms can also be recovered from biopsies of cutaneous lesions. Isolation from these specimens provides more reliable evidence of deep-seated infection than does isolation from broncho-alveolar lavage fluid, sputum or urine.

SEROLOGICAL TESTS

T. beigelii produces a heat-stable antigen which shares antigenic determinants with the capsular antigen of *Cryptococcus neoformans*. A number of reports have appeared indicating that with serum the latex particle agglutination (LPA) test for *C. neoformans* antigen is positive in patients with disseminated trichosporonosis and could be useful in making the diagnosis. However, negative results have also been obtained in LPA tests with serum and urine specimens from patients dying with disseminated trichosporonosis.

27.2.5 Management

Localized deep *Trichosporon* infection in a non-neutropenic patient will often respond to parenteral treatment with amphotericin B (1.0 mg/kg per day). In contrast, in neutropenic individuals, amphotericin B treatment is seldom of benefit unless the neutrophil count recovers. Case reports suggest that fluconazole (400 mg) is often effective in the treatment of trichosporonosis.

27.3 Systemic *Malassezia* infection

Malassezia furfur is the aetiological agent of three forms of mild superficial infection: pityriasis versicolor, *Malassezia* folliculitis and seborrhoeic dermatitis (see Chapter 6). However, this organism can also cause a serious systemic infection in low birth-weight infants and debilitated adults and children who are receiving parenteral lipid nutrition through indwelling vascular catheters. Administration of fat emulsions appears to favour the growth of *M. furfur*, leading to colonization of the catheter and subsequent infection.

27.3.1 Geographical distribution

These infections are worldwide in distribution.

27.3.2   **The causal organism and its habitat**

M. furfur (*Pityrosporum orbiculare, P. ovale*) is a lipophilic yeast which forms part of the normal cutaneous flora of humans. A second species, *Malassezia pachydermatis* has also caused similar systemic infections.

M. furfur catheter-related fungaemia has become a well-recognized complication of total parenteral nutrition (TPN), most cases occurring in infants less than 12 months old. Many of the infants had been born preterm and all required TPN for various underlying disorders. Due to the severe nature of the underlying illness in many of these patients, it is difficult to assess the precise role of *M. furfur* in clinical status and final outcome of patients.

27.3.3   **Clinical manifestations**

In infants, *M. furfur* fungaemia usually presents as fever and/or apnoea and bradycardia. Interstitial pneumonia and thrombocytopenia are common findings in this patient group. The most common symptoms of systemic infection in infants are fever and respiratory distress with or without apnoea. Less frequent symptoms and signs include poor feeding and hepatosplenic enlargement. No signs of infection have been noted at catheter insertion sites, nor has a skin rash been evident in infants with systemic infection.

The few reported adult cases of catheter-associated *M. furfur* sepsis have occurred in conjunction with a range of underlying illnesses. All patients had been receiving parenteral lipid emulsions through central venous catheters for periods ranging from a few days to many months. Fever was the consistent presenting symptom.

The predominant pathological changes noted in patients with catheter-associated *M. furfur* infections have involved the heart and lungs. These have included mycotic thrombi around the tips of indwelling catheters, endocardial vegetations, and inflammatory lesions of the lung.

27.3.4   **Essential investigations and their interpretation**

M. furfur fungaemia has sometimes been diagnosed following detection of the organism in stained smears prepared from catheter blood specimens. However, the diagnosis is most often based on isolation of the organism from blood taken through the catheter. The recovery of *M. furfur* from peripheral blood cultures is poor: the number of organisms isolated is much lower than the number recovered from catheter specimens. Following removal of the catheter, *M. furfur* can often be isolated from the tip.

Although the lipid concentration of conventional broth and agar media is often insufficient to support the growth of *M. furfur*, it would appear that the blood of patients receiving TPN often contains sufficient lipids to permit initial growth of the organism in culture. Subculture of broth onto an agar medium containing, or overlaid with, a lipid source, should ensure isolation of *M. furfur*. Identifiable colonies can be obtained after incubation for 4–6 days at 32°C.

If *M. furfur* sepsis is suspected, the catheter hub (external connecting port) and tip should be cultured in lipid-containing broth.

27.3.5   Management

The most important factor in the successful management of *M. furfur* fungaemia in newborn infants is the removal of the infected vascular catheter, whether or not antifungal treatment is given. Lipid supplements should be discontinued and an antifungal azole, such as parenteral fluconazole (5 mg/kg), should be administered. More stable patients may be able to receive fluconazole or itraconazole by mouth.

Select bibliography

Comprehensive texts

Kibbler, C.C., Mackenzie, D.W.R. & Odds, F.C. (editors) (1996) *Principles and Practice of Clinical Mycology*. John Wiley, Chichester. [This recent textbook contains useful reviews of the clinical manifestations, diagnosis and management of different fungal infections on a systems basis.]

Kwon-Chung, K.J. & Bennett, J.E. (1992) *Medical Mycology*, 4th edn. Lea & Febiger, Philadelphia. [The latest edition of this authoritative textbook covers all aspects of the diagnosis and management of fungal infections.]

Rippon, J.W. (1988) *Medical Mycology. The Pathogenic Fungi and the Pathogenic Actinomycetes*, 3rd edn. WB Saunders, Philadelphia. [Another comprehensive textbook which covers all aspects of fungal and actinomycotic infections.]

Monographs on particular aspects

Elewski, B.E. (editor) (1992) *Cutaneous Fungal Infections*. Igaku-Shoin, New York. [This monograph deals with all aspects of superficial fungal infections and also covers the cutaneous manifestations of systemic infections.]

Hay, R.J. (editor) (1989) *Baillière's Clinical Tropical Medicine and Communicable Diseases: Tropical Fungal Infections*. Baillière Tindall, London. [This monograph remains a useful source of information about the clinical manifestations, diagnosis and management of many of the fungal diseases encountered in the tropics.]

Hay, R.J. (1993) *Fungi and Skin Disease*. Gower Medical Publishing, London. [A concise but informative guide to the diagnosis and management of the different forms of fungal skin disease.]

Meunier, F. (editor) (1995) *Baillière's Clinical Infectious Diseases: Invasive Fungal Infections in Cancer Patients*. Baillière Tindall, London. [This recent monograph contains useful reviews of the clinical manifestations, diagnosis and management of the different fungal diseases encountered in this important group of immunocompromised patients.]

Roberts, D.T., Evans, E.G.V. & Allen, B.R. (1990) *Fungal Nail Infections*. Gower Medical Publishing, London. [A concise but informative guide to the diagnosis and management of onychomycosis.]

Sarosi, G.A. & Davies, S.F. (editors) (1993) *Fungal Diseases of the Lungs*, 2nd edn. Raven Press, New York. [This comprehensive monograph contains much useful information about pulmonary fungal diseases and their aetiological agents, diagnosis and treatment.]

Smith, J.M.B. (1989) *Opportunistic Mycoses of Man and Animals*.

CAB International, Wallingford. [A useful source of information about a number of fungal diseases. Clinical manifestations and management are not covered in detail.]

Warnock, D.W. & Richardson, M.D. (editors) (1991) *Fungal Infection in the Compromised Patient*, 2nd edn. John Wiley, Chichester. [Although some of the treatment recommendations have become outdated, this monograph remains a useful source of information about the clinical manifestations, diagnosis and management of the fungal diseases encountered in AIDS and other groups of immunosuppressed patients.]

Monographs on particular diseases

Bodey, G.P. (editor) (1993) *Candidiasis. Pathogenesis, Diagnosis and Treatment*, 2nd edn. Raven Press, New York. [The latest edition of this monograph contains much useful information about the different clinical forms of candidosis and their diagnosis and treatment.]

Odds, F.C. (1988) *Candida and Candidosis*, 2nd edn. Baillière Tindall, London. [This remains the definitive monograph on all aspects of the organisms and the many different forms of the disease.]

Samaranayake, L.P. & MacFarlane, T.W. (editors) (1990) *Oral Candidosis*. Wright, London. [This well-illustrated monograph contains useful reviews of the clinical manifestations, diagnosis and management of the different clinical forms of this disease.]

Laboratory diagnosis of fungal infection

Chandler, F.W. & Watts, J.C. (1987) *Pathologic Diagnosis of Fungal Infections*. ASCP Press, Chicago. [The excellent colour photographs and descriptions make this an essential reference text.]

Evans, E.G.V. & Richardson, M.D. (editors) (1989) *Medical Mycology: a Practical Approach*. IRL Press at Oxford University Press, Oxford. [Individual contributions contain much useful practical information about the different aspects of laboratory diagnosis of fungal infection.]

Koneman, E.W. & Roberts, G.D. (1985) *Practical Laboratory Mycology*, 3rd edn. Williams & Wilkins, Baltimore. [This illustrated manual describes the different procedures used for processing and culturing of clinical specimens and the identification of organisms. Serological tests are not covered.]

McGinnis, M.R. (1980) *Laboratory Handbook of Medical Mycology*. Academic Press, New York. [Another manual dealing with procedures for processing of specimens and identification of organisms. The excellent illustrations and descriptions make this an essential reference text.]

Salfelder, K. (1990) *Atlas of Fungal Pathology*. Kluwer Academic Publishers, Dordrecht. [Another well-illustrated manual dealing with the histopathological diagnosis of fungal infections.]

Identification manuals

Campbell, C.K., Johnson, E.M., Philpot, C.M. & Warnock, D.W. (1996) *Identification of Pathogenic Fungi*. Public Health Laboratory Service, London. [A well-illustrated guide to the identification of human pathogenic fungi.]

De Hoog, G.S. & Guarro, J. (editors) (1995) *Atlas of Clinical Fungi.* Centraalbureau voor Schimmelcultures, Baarn. [The definitive illustrated guide to the identification of pathogenic fungi.]

Larone, D.H. (1995) *Medically Important Fungi. A Guide to Identification.* 3rd edn. ASM Press, Washington DC. [An illustrated guide to the laboratory identification of fungi.]

St-Germain, G. & Summerbell, R. (1996) *Identifying Filamentous Fungi. A Clinical Laboratory Handbook.* Star Publishing, Belmont. [Another excellent guide to the identification of pathogenic fungi.]

Antifungal chemotherapy

Fernandes, P.B. (editor) (1992) *New Approaches for Antifungal Drugs.* Birkhauser, Boston. [Individual contributions contain much useful information about recent developments in the search for novel antifungal agents.]

Rippon, J.W. & Fromtling, R.A. (editors) (1993) *Cutaneous Antifungal Agents: Selected Compounds in Clinical Practice.* Marcel Dekker, New York. [A useful source of information about the drugs used in the treatment of superficial fungal infections.]

Ryley, J.F. (editor) (1990) *Chemotherapy of Fungal Diseases.* Springer-Verlag, Berlin. [The many excellent contributions to this monograph deal with all aspects of the discovery, development and clinical use of antifungal drugs. Although some of the treatment recommendations have become outdated, it remains a most useful source of information.]

Introductory texts

Clayton, Y.M. & Midgley, G. (1985) *Medical Mycology. Pocket Picture Guide.* Gower Medical, London. [A short illustrated introduction to the subject with brief descriptions of diagnostic procedures.]

Evans, E.G.V. & Gentles, J.C. (1985) *Essentials of Medical Mycology.* Churchill Livingstone, Edinburgh. [This text is recommended as a clear and concise introduction to the subject. Management of patients is not discussed in detail.]

Recommended reviews

Bennett, J.E., Hay, R.J. & Peterson, P.K. (editors) (1992) *New Strategies in Fungal Disease.* Churchill Livingstone, Edinburgh.

Borgers, M., Hay, R.J. & Rinaldi, M.G. (editors) (1992) *Current Topics in Medical Mycology*, Vol. 4. Springer Verlag, New York.

Borgers, M., Hay, R.J. & Rinaldi, M.G. (editors) (1992) *Current Topics in Medical Mycology*, Vol. 5. Prous Science Publishers, Barcelona.

Jacobs, P.H. & Nall, L. (editors) (1996) *Fungal Disease. Biology, Immunology and Diagnosis.* Marcel Dekker, New York.

Vanden Bossche, H., Odds, F.C. & Kerridge, D. (editors) (1993) *Dimorphic Fungi in Biology and Medicine.* Plenum Press, New York.

Index

Abelcet (ABLC) 20
    adverse reactions 29–30
    in crytococcosis 157–8
    in disseminated candidosis 143,
        146
    in *Fusarium* infection 219
    mode of administration 27–8
    in mucormycosis 165
    pharmaceutics 24
    pharmacokinetics 22
    therapeutic use 24–5
Absidia corymbifera, infection by,
        see mucormycosis
acquired immune deficiency
        syndrome (AIDS) 1, 3, 6–7
    and blastomycosis 169–70
    and candidosis 132, 139–40,
        142
    and coccidiodomycosis 174,
        175–6
    and cryptococcosis 149, 151,
        152, 153–4, 155, 157–8
    and histoplasmosis 186–7
    and *Penicillium marneffei*
        infection 223–6
    and phaeohyphomycosis 229
    and sporotrichosis 216
    and trichosporonosis 233
Acremonium spp., infection by 104
acute pseudomembranous
        candidosis (thrush) 79
Alternaria spp., infection by, *see*
        phaeohyphomycosis
AmBisome 20
    adverse reactions 29–30
    in cryptococcosis, AIDS
        patients 157
    in disseminated candidosis 143,
        146
    in *Fusarium* infection 219
    in invasive aspergillosis 126, 127
    metabolism 23
    mode of administraation 27–28
    in mucormycosis 165
    pharmaceutics 23
    pharmacokinetics 22–3
    therapeutic use 24
amorolfine 52
    in onychomycosis 92, 106
Amphocil (Amphotec, ABCD) 20
    adverse reactions 29–30
    in cryptococcosis 157–8

in disseminated candidosis 143,
        146
in *Fusarium* infection 219
mode of administration 22
in mucormycosis 165
pharmaceutics 24
pharmacokinetics 22–3
therapeutic use 245
amphotericin
    adverse reactions 20, 28–9
    in aspergillosis 125, 128, 129,
        130
    in blastomycosis 171
    in chromoblastomycosis 197
    in coccidioidomycosis 179, 180
    in cryptococcosis 156–9
    in deep candidosis 142–8
    in *Fusarium* infection 219
    in hepatosplenic
        candidosis 147–48
    in histoplasmosis 189–90
    interaction with other drugs 30
    in keratomycosis 109
    laboratory monitoring 55–6
    lipid-based formulations 20, *see*
        also named agents
    in *Malassezia furfur* catheter-
        related fungaemia 236
    mechanism of action 20–1
    metabolism 23
    mode of administration 25–7
    in mucormycosis 165–6
    in oral candidosis 87–8, 89
    oral suspension, as
        prophylaxis 54
    in otomycosis 112
    in paracoccidioidomycosis 194
    in *Penicillium marneffei*
        infection 225
    in phaeohyphomycosis 231
    pharmaceutics 23
    pharmacokinetics 21–2
    resistance to 21, 222
    in *Scedosporium* infection 222
    spectrum of action 21
    in sporotrichosis 216
    in superficial candidosis 88
    therapeutic use 24–5
    in trichosporonosis 234
angular cheilitis 80
antifungals
    empirical usage 53–4

laboratory monitoring 55–8
prophylactic usage 54–5
see also named agents
arthritis, due to
Blastomyces dermatitidis 168–9
Candida spp. 137–8
Coccidioides immitis 175
Histoplasma spp. 186
paracoccidioidomycosis 193
Penicillium marneffei 224
Scedosporium sp. 221
Sporothrix schenkii 214
aspergilloma 115, 125
aspergillosis
acute invasive 116–17, 125–8
and AIDS 121–2
allergic 114–15, 124–5
aspergilloma 115, 125
causal organisms 113
cerebral 118–19, 129
chronic necrotising of
lung 115–16, 125
cutaneous 120–1, 130
empirical treatment 127
endocarditis 119–20, 129
gastrointestinal 121
hepatosplenic 121
laboratory investigations 122–4
management 124–30
myocarditis 119–20
nosocomial 113
obstructing bronchial 117, 128
ocular 107–110, 119, 129
onychomycosis 104–6
osteomyelitis 120, 129
otomycosis 111–2
paranasal sinuses 117–18, 128
tracheobronchitis 117, 128
Aspergillus spp., infection by, *see*
aspergillosis
azole antifungals, *see named drugs*

basidiobolomycosis 199–201
Basidobolus ranarum, infection by,
see basidiobolomycosis
bifonazole 52, 96
Bipolaris spp., infection by, *see*
phaeohyphomycosis
black piedra 100–1
Blastomyces dermatitidis, infection
by, *see* blastomycosis
blastomycosis
and AIDS 169–70
causal organism 167
cutaneous 168
disseminated 169
genitourinary 169
laboratory investigations 170–1
management 171
meningitis 169

osteoarticular 168–69
pulmonary 168
Blastoschizomyces capitatus
(Trichosporon capitatum),
infection by, *see*
trichosporonosis
blood, collection and culture
of 12–13
bone
aspergillosis of 118, 120
blastomycosis of 168–9
candidosis of 136–7
coccidioidomycosis of 175
cryptococcosis of 152–3
mycetoma of 206
mucormycosis of 161–2
Scedosporium infection of 220
sporotrichosis of 213–4
bone marrow, collection 14
bone marrow transplantation 6
aspergillosis in 113, 117, 118,
119
fusarium infection in 218
trichosporonosis in 233
brain
aspergillosis of 118–19
blastomycosis of 169
candidosis of 133–4
coccidioldomycosis of 175
cryptococcosis of 151–2
histoplasmosis of 185
mucormycosis of 161, 162–3
paracoccidiodomycosis of 193
phaeohyphomycosis of 229
broncheolar lavage specimens,
collection 14
burns, and mucormycosis 163

Candida, spp.
infection by, *see* candidosis
isolation from human host 3,
131
in tinea unguium 84–5
Candida albicans
infection by, *see* candidosis
isolation from human host 78–9
resistance to azoles 86
resistance to flucytosine 36
Candida (Tonrulopsis) glabrata,
resistance to
fluconazole 131
Candida guilliermondii 78
Candida krusei, resistance to
fluconazole 131
Candids lusitaniae, resistance to
amphotericin 21
Candida parapsilosis, and
paronychia 84
Candida tropicalis, in
otomycosis 111

Candidaemia 137–8, 146–7
candidosis
    acute disseminated 138, 146–7
    and AIDS 79, 88, 132, 139–40
    arthritis 137, 145
    balanitis 82–3, 91
    central nervous system 133–4
    chronic disseminated 138–9,
        147–8
    chronic mucocutaneous 85–6,
        92–3
    congenital cutaneous 84
    cutaneous 83–4, 92
    empirical treatment 147
    endocarditis 134, 143
    endophthalmitis 137, 145–6
    gastric 133
    hepatosplenic 138–9, 147–8
    in heroin addicts 139
    and intensive care 132
    intertrigo 83
    intrauterine 136
    laboratory investigations 87, 140
    and leucoplakia 79
    in low-birth-weight infants 139
    of lung 133
    meningitis 133–4, 143
    myocarditis 134–5
    myositis 136–7
    of nail 74, 84–5, 92
    oesophageal 132, 142–3
    oral 79–81
    osteomyelitis 136, 145
    pericarditis 135
    peritonitis 136, 144–5
    otomycosis 111
    renal 135, 144
    and thrombosis 143
    and tinea pedis 83
    of urinary tract 135, 144
    vaginal 81–2, 89–91
candiduria 135–6
central nervous system
    aspergillosis of 119
    blastomycosis of 169
    candidosis of 133–4
    coccidioidomycosis of 175
    cryptococcosis of 151–2
    histoplasmosis of 185
    mucormycosis of 163
    phaeohyphomycosis of 229
chest fluids, collection 14
chromoblastomycosis
    (chromomycosis) 195–97
chromomycosis, see
        chromoblastomycosis
chronic granulomatous disease, and
        aspergillosis 114, 116
Cladosporium carrionii, infection
        by, see chromoblastomycosis

clotrimazole 52
    in superficial candidosis 90, 91
    in dermatophytosis 66, 68, 71,
        74
    in keratomycosis 109
    in otomycosis 112
    in pityriasis versicolor 96
Coccidioides immitis, infection by,
        see coccidioidomycosis
coccidioidomycosis
    and AIDS 175–6
    chronic 173–4
    disseminated 174–5, 180
    laboratory investigations 176–8
    management 178–81
    meningitis 175, 180–1
    pulmonary 173–4, 178–80
combination therapy, of antifungal
        agents, see named drugs
Conidiobolus coronatus, infection
        by, see conidiobolomycosis,
        rhinofacial
conidiobolomycosis,
        rhinofacial 198–99
co-trimoxazole, in
        actinomycetoma 208
cornea, see keratomycosis
cryptococcosis
    and AIDS 149, 150, 151, 152,
        153–4
    cutaneous 152, 159
    disseminated 150
    laboratory investigations 154–6
    management 156–9
    meningitis 151–2, 156
    ocular 153
    osteomyelitis 152–3
    prostatic 153
    pulmonary 150–1, 158–9
Cryptococcus neoformans
infection by, see cryptococcosis
Cryptococcosis neoformans var.
        gattii, infection by, see
        cryptococcosis
Cunninghamella bertholletiae,
        infection by, see
        mucormycosis
cutaneous lesions
    in aspergillosis 120–1
    in blastomycosis 168
    in candidosis 83–4, 139
    in chromoblastomycosis 195–6
    in coccidioidomycosis 173, 175
    in cryptococcosis 152
    in dermatophytusis, see named
        diseases
    in fusarium infection 218
    in histoplasmosis 186
    in lobomycosis 202–3
    in mucormycosis 163

in paracoccidioidomycosis 192
in *Penicillium marneffei*
  infection 224
in sporotrichosis 213
in trichosporonosis 233
Curvularia spp.
  infection by, *see*
    phaeohyphomycosis
  in keratomycosis 107
cyclosporin, interaction with
  azoles 35, 44

dandruff, and *Malassezia
  furfur* 97
dapsone, in actinomycotina 208
denture stomatitis 80
dermatophyte fungi, *see named
  fungi and diseases*
dermatophytosis
  causal organisms 59–60
  laboratory investigations 60–1
  and specimen collection 10–11,
    60
  see also named diseases
diabetes mellitus
  and mucormycosis 161

ear, *see* otomycosis
econazole
  in dermatophytosis 66, 68, 71,
    74
  in keratomycosis 109
  in otomycosis 112
  in pityriasis versicolor 96
  in superficial candidosis 90–1
endocarditis, due to
  Aspergillus spp. 119–20
  Candida spp. 134–5
endophthalmitis, due to
  Aspergillus spp. 119
  Candida spp. 137
  Sporothrix schenkii 214
  Trichosporon beigelii 232
entomophthoramycosis
  basidiobolomycosis 199–201
  rhinofacial
    conidiobolomycosis 198–9
Epidermophyton floccosum,
  infection by 65, 67, 69, 72
Eye
  collection of specimens 12,
    108–9
  see also endophthalmitis;
    keratomycosis
Exophiala spp., infection by, *see*
  phaeohyphomycosis
Exserohilum spp., infection by, *see*
  phaeohyphomycosis

favus 634

fluconazole
  adverse reactions to 34
  in blastomycosis 171
  in chronic mucocutaneous
    candidosis 93
  in coccidioidomycosis 179–81
  in cryptococcal meningitis 157
  in disseminated candidosis 142,
    143, 144, 145, 146–7
  in hepatosplenic candidosis 148
  interaction with other
    drugs 34–5
  in keratomycosis 110
  laboratory monitoring 56
  mechanism of action 30
  metabolism 32
  mode of administration 33–4
  in oesophagitis, candida 142–3
  in oral candidosis 88–9
  in paracoccidioidomycosis 194
  pharmaceutics 32
  pharmacokinetics 31–2
  as prophylaxis 55, 147
  resistance to 31, 89
  spectrum of action 30–1
  in sporotrichosis 215
  therapeutic use 32–3
  in vaginal candidosis 90, 91
flucytosine
  adverse reaction to 37
  in chromoblastomycosis 197
  in cryptococcosis 156
  in disseminated candidosis 143,
    147
  interaction with other drugs 38
  laboratory monitoring 57
  mechanism of action 35
  metaolism 36
  mode of administration 37, 38
  pharmaceutics 37
  pharmacokinetics 36
  resistance to 36
  spectrum of action 35
  therapeutic use 37
5-fluorocytosine, *see* flucytosine
Fonsecaea spp., infection by, *see*
  chromoblastomycosis
fungaemia, due to
  Aspergillus spp. 123
  Candida spp. 137–8
  Fusarium spp. 218
  Malassezia furfur 235–6
Fusarium spp., infection by
  disseminated 217–20
  keratomycosis 107
  onychomycosis 104–6

gastrointestinal tract
  aspergillosis of 121
  candidosis of 133

histoplasmosis of 186
mucormycosis of 162–3
genitourinary tract
blastomycosis of 169
candidosis of 144
cryptococcosis of 153
griseofulvin
adverse reaction to 40
in dermatophytosis 67, 68, 77
interaction with other drugs 40
mechanism of action 38–9
metabolism 39
pharmaceutics 39
pharmacokinetics 39
in pityriasis versicolor 96
resistance to 39
spectrum of action 39
therapeutic use 39–40

heart
aspergillosis of 119–20
candidosis of 134–5
histoplasmosis of 185
trichosporonosis of 232
heart transplantation
and aspergillosis 119–20
and candidosis 132
Hendersonula toruloidea, see
Scytalidium dimidiatum
Histoplasma capsulatum, infection
by, *see* histoplasmosis
Histoplasmosis duboisii, infection
by, *see* histoplasmosis
histoplasmosis
acute pulmonary 183–4, 189
African 186
and AIDS 186–7
causal organisms 182–3
chronic pulmonary 184, 189
disseminated 185–6, 190
laboratory investigations 187–9
management 189–90
human immune deficiency virus,
infection by, *see* acquired
immune deficiency (AIDS)
hyalohyphomycosis 217–22, *see*
also named infections

imidazole antifungals, *see named*
agents
itraconazole
in acute invasive
aspergillosis 125–8
adverse reactions 43
in aspergillus osteomyelitis 129
in aspergillus sinusitis 117–18
in blastomycosis 171
in candida onychomycosis 92
in chromoblastomycosis 197

in chronic mucocutaneous
candidosis 93
in chronic necrotising
aspergillosis 125
in coccidiomycosis 180, 181
in cryptococcal meningitis 157
in dermatophytosis 67, 68, 72,
77
in disseminated candidosis 147
in fusarium infection 220
in histoplasmosis 189, 190
interaction with other drugs 44
in keratomycosis 110
laboratory monitoring 578
mechanism of action 40–1
metabolism 42
mode of administration 42–3
in mycetoma 209
in obstructing bronchial
aspergillosis 128
in onychomycosis 106
in oral candidosis 89
in paracoccioidomycosis 194
in paranasal sinus
aspergillosis 128
in *Penicillium marneffei*
infection 225, 226
in phaeohyphomycosis 231
pharmaceutics 42
pharmacokinetics 41–2
in pityriasis versicolor 96
as prophylaxis 147
resistance to 41
in rhinofacial
conidiobolomycosis 199
in *Scedosporium* infection 222
spectrum of action 41
in sporotrichosis 215, 216
therapeutic use 42
in tracheobronchitis 128
in vaginal candidosis 90
isoconazole nitrate 53
in vaginal candidosis 90

joints, infection of, *see* arthritis

keratomycosis 107–10
ketoconazole
administration 46
adverse reactions 46–7
in basidiobolomycosis 199
in blastomycosis 171
in coccidioidomycosis 179, 180
in chronic mucocutaneous
candidosis 93
in histoplasmosis 189
interaction with other drugs 47
in keratomycosis 110
in mycetoma 209
laboratory monitoring 58

mechanism of action 45
metabolism 45
mode of administration 46
in oesophagitis, candida 142
in oral candidosis 88
in paracoccidioidomycosis 194
in *Penicillium marneffei*
    infection 225
pharmaceutics 45
pharmacokinetics 45
in pityriasis versicolor 96
prophylaxis 54
resistance to 45
in rhinofacial
    conidiobolomycosis 199
in *Scedosporium* infection 222
in seborrhoeic dermatitis 98
spectrum of action 45
kidney
    candidosis of 135
    trichosporonosis of 233

leukaemia
    and aspergillosis 114, 125–6
    and candidosis 138
    and fusarium infection 218
    and trichosporonosis 233
liposomal amphotericin B, *see*
    AmBisome
liver
    aspergillosis of 121
    candidosis of 138–9
    coccidioidomycosis of 175
    cryptococcosis of 153
    histoplasmosis of 185
    paracoccidioidomycosis of 193
Loboa loboi, infection by, *see*
    lobomycosis
lobomycosis 202–3
low-birth-weight infants
    and candidosis 139
    and *Malassezia furfur*
        infection 235
lower respiratory tract, collection of
    specimens 13–14
lung
    aspergillosis of 114–22, 124–28
    blastomycosis of 168
    candidosis of 133
    coccidioidomycosis of 173–4
    cryptococcosis of 150–1
    fusarium infection of 218
    histoplasmosis of 183–5
    Malassezia furfur infection
        of 235
    mucormycosis of 162
    paracoccidioidomycosis of 192
    Penicillium marneffei infection
        of 224
    Scedosprium infection of 220–1

sporotrichosis of 214
trichosporonosis of 233

Madurella mycetomatis, infection
    by, *see* mycetoma
magnetic resonance, in diagnosis of
    fungal infection 119
Malassezia furfur, infection by
    catheter-related
        fungaemia 234–36
    folliculitis 97
    pityriasis versicolor 94–6
    in seborrhoeic dermatitis 97–8
Meningitis, due to
    aspergillosis 119
    blastomycosis 169
    candidosis 133–4, 143
    coccidioidomycosis 175
    cryptococcosis 151–2
    histoplasmosis 185
    mucormycosis 163
    phaeohyphomycosis 229
miconazole
    adverse reaction to 49
    in dermatophytosis 66, 68, 71,
        74
    in keratomycosis 109
    interaction with other drugs 50
    mechanism of action 47–8
    metabolism 48
    pharmaceutics 48
    pharmacokinetics 48
    in pityriasis versicolor 96
    resistance to 48
    in *Scedosporium* infection 222
    spectrum of action 48
    in superficial candidosis 90, 91
    therapeutic use 49
Microsporum audouinii, in tinea
    capitis 62, 63
Microsporum canis, infection
    by 61, 63, 65, 72
Miccrosporum equinum, in tinea
    capitis 62
Microsporum ferrugineum, in tinea
    capitis 62
Microsporum gypseum, infection
    by 72
Mucor spp.
    in otomycosis 111
    other infections, *see*
        mucormycosis
mucormycosis
    cerebral 161–2
    cutaneous 163
    disseminated 163
    endocarditis 164
    gastrointestinal 162–3
    laboratory investigations 164
    management 165–6

pulmonary 162
rhinocerebral 161–2
mycetoma
    laboratory investigations 207–8
    management 208–9
mycotic keratitis, see keratomycosis
myocarditis, due to
    Aspergillus spp. 119–20
    Candida spp. 134–5

naftifine 53, 66, 68, 71, 74
nail
    candidosis of 74, 75
    collection 10–11
    dermatophytosis of 74–7
    mould infection of 76, 104–6
natamycin 53
    in keratomycosis 109
    in otomycosis 112
nystatin 53
    in candidosis 87–8, 90, 91, 92
    in otomycosis 112

oesophagus
    candidosis of 132–3
    and AIDS 32–3, 139–40, 142–3
onychomycosis, see nail
oral leukoplakia, and
        candidosis 79, 88
osteomyelitis, see bone
otomycosis 111–12

Paecilomyces spp., infection
        by 222
Paracoccidioides *brasiliensis*,
        infection by, see
        paracoccidioidomycosis
paracoccidioidomycosis
    causal organism 191
    disseminated 193
    laboratory investigations 193–4
    lymphonodular 193
    management 194
    mucocutaneous 192–3
    pulmonary 191–2
parenteral nutrition, and
        Malassezia furfur
        infection 234–6
Penicillium spp.
    in keratomycosis 107
    in otomcosis 111
Penicllium marneffei, infection
        by 7, 223–6
pericarditis, see heart
peritoneal dialysis
    and candidosis 136
    and trichosporonosis 232
*Phaeoannellomyces werneckii
        (Exophiala werneckii)*, in
        tinea nigra 101

phaeohyphomycosis 227–31
    cerebral 229
    cutaneous 229
    laboratory investigations 230
    management 231
    paranasal sinus 228
    subcutaneous 228
Phialophora spp., infection by, see
        phaeohyphomycosis
Phialophora verrucosa, infection
        by, see
        chromoblastomycosis
phycomycosis, see mucormycosis
piedra 98, see also black piedra;
        white piedra
Piedra hortae, in black piedra 100
pityriasis versicolor 94–6
*Pityrosporum orbiculare, see
        Malassezia furfur*
*Pityrosporum ovale, see Malassezia
        furfur*
polyene antifungals, see *named
        agents*
potassium iodide
    in basidiobolomycosis 200–1
    in rhinofacial
        conidiobolomycosis 199
    in sporotrichosis 215–6
prednisone, in allergic
        aspergillosis 124
prophylaxis 54–5
    see also named *mycoses*
prostate, cryptococcosis of 153
*Pseudallescheria boydii, see
        Scedosporium
        apiospermum*
pus, collection 14
pyelonephritis, see kidney,
        cryptococcosis of

Ramichloridium cerophilum,
        infection by, see
        chromoblastomycosis
Rhinocladiella acquaspersa,
        infection by, see
        chromoblastomycosis
rhinosporidiosis 210–11
Rhinosporidium seeberi, infection
        by, see rhinosporidiosis
Rhizomucor pusillus, infection by,
        see mucormycosis
Rhizopus spp., in otomycosis 111
*Rhizopus arrhizus
        (Rhizopus oryzae)*, infection
        by, see mucormycosis
Rhizopus oryzae, infection by, see
        mucormycosis
Rhizopus rhizopodiformis,
        infection by, see
        mucormycosis

rifampicin, in actinomycetoma 208

Sakesenaea vasiformis, infection by, *see* mucormycosis
Scedosporium apiospermum, infection by 220–2
Scedosporium prolificans , infection by 220–2
Scopulariopsis brevicaulis, infection by 104–6, 222
Scytalidium dimidiatum, infection by 71, 102
Scytalidium *hyalinum*, infection by 71, 102
seborrhoeic dermatitis 97–8
selenium sulphide, in pityriasis versicolor 96
serological tests
    specimen collection 15
    see also individual diseases
skin
    collection 10–11
    see cutaneous lesions; *and named mycoses*
sinus
    aspergillosis of 114, 117–18
    mucormycosis of 161
    phaeohyphomycosis of 228–9
    rhinofacial conidiobolomycosis of 198
    rhinosporidiosis of 210–11
spleen
    aspergillosis of 121
    candidosis of 138–9, 147–8
    histoplasmosis of 186
    Penicillium marneffei infection of 224
sporotrichosis
    causal organism 212
    cutaneous 213
    extracutaneous 213–14
    laboratory investigations 215
    management 215–16
Sporothrix schenckii, infection by, *see* sporotrichosis
streptomycin sulphate, in actinomycetoma 208
sulconazole 53
    in dermatophytosis 66, 68, 71, 74
    in pityriasis versicolor 96
sulphadiazine, in paracocidioidomycosis 194
sulphadoxine-pyrimethamine, in actinomycetoma 209

terbinafine
    adverse reactions to 52
    in candidosis 92
    in dermatophytosis 66, 67, 68, 71, 72, 74, 77

interaction with other drugs 52
    mechanism of action 50
    metabolism 51
    mode of administration 51
    pharmaceutics 51
    pharmacokinetics 50–1
    in pityriasis versicolor 96
    resistance to 50
    spectrum of action 50
    therapeutic use 51
thiabendazole, in chromoblastomycosis 197
tinea capitis 61–5
tinea corporis 65–7
tinea cruris 67–9
tinea manuum 72–4
tinea nigra 101–2
tinea pedis 69–72
tinea unguium 74–7
tinea versocolor, *see* pityriasis versicolor
thrush, *see* candidosis
tissue, collection 13
tioconazole 53, 77
    in tinea unguium 77
Trichophyton mentagrophytes, infection by 62
Trichophyton mentagrophytes var. *interdigitale*, infection by 69, 72, 74
Trichophyton rubrum, infection by 67, 69, 72, 74
Trichophyton tonsurans, infection by 61, 65
Trichophyton soudanense, in tinea capitis 62
Trichophyton schoenleinii, in tinea capitis 62, 63
Trichophyton verrucosum, infection by 62, 65, 72
Trichophyton violaceum, in tinea capitis 62
Trichosporon beigelii, infection by, *see* trichosporonosis; white piedra
Trichosporon capitatum, infection by, see trichosporonosis
trichosporonosis 232–4, *see also* white piedra

urinary tract
    candidosis of 135–6, 144
    cryptococcosis of 153
    trichosporonosis of 232
urine, collection 13

vagina, secretion, specimen collection 11
vascular catheterization, and fungal infection

and candidosis 137–8
Malassezia furfur 234–6

white piedra 98–100
Wood's light
  dermatophytosis 11, 63
  and diagnosis 11

in pityriasis versicolor 95
in tinea capitis 63
Xylohypha (Cladophialophora)
    bantiana, infection by, *see*
    phaeohyphomycosis

zygomycosis, *see* mucormycosis